1 (919) 872-5929

Hurry Up and Rest!

AL CADENHEAD, JR.

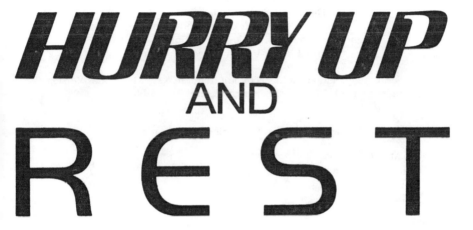

HURRY UP AND REST

BROADMAN PRESS
Nashville, Tennessee

© Copyright 1988 • Broadman Press
All rights reserved
4254-38

ISBN: 0-8054-5438-1
Dewey Decimal Classification: 613.7
Subject Heading: REST
Library of Congress Catalog Card Number: 88-19809
Printed in the United States of America

The Scripture quotations in this book are from the New King James Version.
Copyright © 1979, 1980, 1982, Thomas Nelson, Inc., Publishers.

Library of Congress Cataloging-in-Publication Data

Cadenhead, Al, 1947-
  Hurry up and rest! / Al Cadenhead, Jr.
     p.   cm.
  ISBN 0-8054-5438-1
  1. Rest.   I.Title.
RA785.C34 1989
613.7'9—dc19   88-19809

To Suzanne

Acknowledgments

Before we begin this brief journey together, allow me the opportunity to thank some of the special people who made this book possible. I am indebted, first of all, to Broadman for their confidence in allowing me to author a second book for them.

Since the scope of this book exceeded the normal range of pastoral duties, I had to depend on guidance from special friends in the medical field. I sincerely thank Dr. Rob DuRant, Dr. Wayne Hodges, Dr. Julius Johnson, and Dr. Charles Shaefer for their concern and consultation. As a longtime student of Dr. Wayne Oates, I am honored by his writing the foreword for this book.

Writing is a therapeutic process for me, but not always for the one who must turn unfinished sentences and omitted words into a presentable manuscript. My thanks, therefore, go to my secretary, Mrs. Wyanne Hall, for "hanging in there."

To my family and friends whose prayers are reality, thanks.

Foreword

Dr. Cadenhead speaks convincingly and helpfully to one of the most difficult audiences to whom to write: those who are hurried and harried, restless and driven by both the real and the imagined tasks they have to do. He may, for example, hear some of these people say: "I had a member of my family give me a copy of your book, but I have not had time to read it!" He may be called by a family member of some loved one in a coronary care unit. The family may have been trying for months to get the patient to slow down, to get enough sleep, to take a day off, to "take care of himself." Yet none of this was to any avail. Now this loved one has had a heart attack. A family member *has* read Dr. Cadenhead's book and wants him to visit the loved one in the coronary care unit!

If you are harassed, driven, and exhausted, read this book *now* yourself! Do not wait for a family member of yours to call either the book to your attention or send Dr. Cadenhead to see you in a coronary care unit!

Dr. Cadenhead does not speak to you as detached, uninvolved observer of persons for whom rest is a lost art and a peripheral priority. He begins the book and continues the discussion with personal dilemmas of his own in squeezing and teasing out of a busy schedule time for the renewal that only God's gift of rest and sleep will give.

In addition, this book encompasses dependable reporting on the work of physicians who are concerned not only with fighting disease but also with teaching us the functions of rest and sleep in keeping us well and in preventing disease. Yet, these reports are presented in a nontechnical manner that informs accurately without intimidating the reader with technical jargon. The author has done careful research and has consulted with specialists on his subject matter.

Especially fascinating to me is the chapter on the way the teachings of Luther and Calvin on the cleansing and sustaining power of work has been secularized and perverted into commercialism and consumerism to the neglect and exhaustion of persons in meaningless work and fretful consumerism. He lays the axe to the root of the tree that bears the bitter fruit of restless fatigue. As Wordsworth said:

> The world is too much with us; late and soon,
> Getting and spending, we lay waste our powers;
> ....
> For this, for everything, we are out of tune.

Our times are, indeed, out of joint, out of tune, and out of synchrony with the way in which God made us.

Al Cadenhead asks for an agonizing reappraisal, not just of our use of time and practice of rest, but also of our basic spiritual relationship to God, to ourselves, to our loved ones, and to our work associates.

WAYNE E. OATES, Ph.D.
Professor of Psychiatry and Behavioral Sciences
School of Medicine, University of Louisville
Louisville, Kentucky

Preface

The great football coach Vince Lombardi once said, "Fatigue makes cowards of us all." In making such a statement he was pointing to the simple truth that we cannot be at our best when we do not provide adequate opportunities of rest for ourselves. Our cowardice does not necessarily take the form of the lack of courage. Instead, we may discover that we simply cannot do what is demanded of us. The result is a great deal of frustration and guilt. The willingness and desire may be genuine, but we just can't produce! We also may discover that our struggle for rest is a spiritual journey.

Most of us have, at some point, learned a similar lesson from our experience with automobiles. If we properly maintain our vehicles, they will usually provide satisfactory service. Yet, ignore some common sense principles and drive an automobile too hard, too long, and disregard regular servicing and the vehicle will operate dependably for only a very brief period of time. Even worse, the vehicle will usually pick a most inappropriate time and place to break down. There can be little question, however, that a breakdown is inevitable. Routine maintenance cannot be ignored.

Why can we readily accept such a fact about an automobile and ignore the truth about ourselves? Too many of us appear to operate under the assumption that we can treat our bodies any way we choose and continue to function productively amid the normal demands of everyday living.

In my daily work I am privileged to have opportunities to hear the true feelings of many people. Frequently I hear the expressions of frustration, guilt, and a loss of joy in life from "fellow travelers." These feelings do not always occur as a result of some great crisis but during the normal routine of one's life. Too many people are trying to produce in the midst of routine exhaustion.

A simple observation of nature will underscore the rhythm of work and rest. Yet, true rest is not as simple as it might appear. We usually equate rest with inactivity. Nothing could be further from the truth. True rest is so much more than the absence of life's hustle and bustle.

The pages of this book are a product of my own, sometimes selfish, concern. I share this labor out of my own struggle and my observation of people all around me. The issue of rest has been a journey for me, and I am not finished yet. Some of my lessons have been very expensive, just as many of yours have been. I am still traveling and I ask you to join me on the journey.

Contents

1

A Personal Dilemma

For Father's Day my family really came through. Instead of the traditional tie and socks, the package was long and rather heavy. The gift came as a result of hints I had given for weeks. They finally gave me a rope hammock. I had seen hammocks in several backyards, and a hammock appeared to me to be the epitome of rest and relaxation.

I found two big pine trees in my backyard that were just the right distance apart for me to hang my new symbol of rest. To lie in a hammock really is a heavenly experience. The ropes go with the contour of the body and create a very pleasant feeling of suspension.

To make the experience even better I tied another rope to a camellia bush a few feet away so that I could pull against the rope while lying in the hammock and swing with practically no effort at all. There are few places more peaceful than this particular spot in my backyard. The pine trees are tall and make a soothing sound as the wind blows through them. A fence frames the yard, and the house conveniently blocks all view from the street. From the very beginning of this experience, I promised myself that I would make use of this new status symbol. I envisioned every evening coming to a close with me swinging and enjoying the sky above.

A couple of years have passed and I must now acknowledge that I have made some use of my family's gift but most of the time the hammock hangs very lonely in the backyard. Now it symbolizes not a place of rest but a sense of failure in another one of those good intentions never quite realized.

From the beginning let me say that my dilemma comes not because of my own importance nor abnormal demands placed upon my life. I have no more responsibility than any one else who takes his or her profession seriously. So, I cannot blame my poor discipline of rest on external demands. The problem is much deeper and considerably more personal.

Some other experiences in my life have become symbolic of my futile attempts to learn how to rest and relax. For example, I have tried to make better use of Saturdays as a day to relax and rest. Saturdays have always been special days for me. I have found Sundays to be anything but days of leisure. My wife is an elementary school teacher. Combine my schedule, hers, and that of our school-age children and the result is typically hectic routine. Therefore, I live from Saturday to Saturday with the goal of making this day a time to relax. Notice that I used the word *goal*. I have visions of how Saturdays are supposed to be. In fact, I occasionally see people who look like they have mastered Saturdays. They are dressed in jogging suits and clean running shoes and obviously they are resting. They probably slept late, ate a leisurely breakfast, read the newspaper, and then napped during the afternoon ball game on television.

I am positive that somewhere there are people who have restful Saturdays. Every week my intentions are to make it work out so that I have that kind of day. On several occasions I have cut my lawn at night during the week so that I would not have to do it on Saturday. My neighbors think I am strange, but they don't understand. They just don't realize I am doing all of this so I can rest on Saturday and have a nice, relaxing day and wear my jogging suit and running shoes.

One point at which my neighbors really questioned my mental health was the night I decided that, if I could get the shutters painted on the front of my house, I could have all day Saturday to wear my jogging suit and lie in my hammock. So I brought out my long extension cord and a light and painted my shutters between 11:00 PM and 1:00 AM. A couple of weeks later my next-door neighbor handled the matter very well when she said that she noticed I had really been working hard on the house. She added, "You are really energetic to be painting at night." She was too kind to say what she was really thinking, *What is wrong with you? Nobody paints the outside of a house at night!*

But, you see, she did not understand my motivation. I was getting everything caught up so that I could rest on Saturday. My jogging suit and hammock were going to be waiting for me on Saturday. By the way, the shutters didn't look bad to have been painted at midnight. I have to admit that it was a bit comical to watch people drive by and try to figure out what someone was doing on a ladder in front of the house, holding a paintbrush in one hand and an electric light in the other, while balancing a gallon paint bucket on top of the ladder. Cars would slow

down, but I could not see the drivers' faces in the dark-
ness. I imagine they were questioning the stability of this
relatively new homeowner in the neighborhood.

But, you see, they just did not understand that I was
getting it all done so that I could rest on Saturday. On
Saturday I was going to take a deep breath and rest all day
long. In fact I probably would plan a brief trip on Saturday
to the mall and wear my jogging suit so that everybody
could look at me an say to themselves, *Here is a guy who
has it under control.* In fact, I have an almost new pair of
running shoes in my closet that I save to wear when I can
look relaxed on Saturday afternoon.

Yet, I must confess that my running shoes are seldom
worn. That presents another problem. My wife gave me
those shoes for Christmas, and she is a bit sensitive that I
don't wear them often. She doesn't understand that I am
saving them for leisurely Saturdays like other people
have.

The problem is that leisurely Saturdays seldom ever
come around. In spite of my best efforts, something often
needs to be done and the leisure hours seldom become
reality. Circumstances invariably provide some kind of
demand. Most of these demands are important, but they
still require energy and time, commodities which most of
us have not accepted as limited resources.

The dilemma is much more complex than the issue of
Saturdays. Saturday is just one of the more obvious points
of frustration. And to be honest, when times of physical
inactivity roll around there is no guarantee of rest. Our
mental, emotional, and spiritual dimensions must cooperate with the physical if true rest is going to take place.

Most of us can think of times when we were physically
inactive, but we were not at all close to any state of rest.
The discipline of rest requires cooperation of our physical,

mental, emotional, and spiritual dimensions. Rest is so much more than just physical inactivity.

For a long time the issue of rest and relaxation has been a concern of mine. If I believed this matter to be unique to me, I would reserve my concern for my mentors and make my confession very private. Unless I am badly mistaken, the issue of rest is a concern of many people today. The problem is much deeper and more serious than Saturdays not turning out exactly right. The problem is complex and deep, and there are few simple answers.

The last thing in the world I want is to become lazy and unproductive. To the depths of my being I believe we were designed by God with creative abilities. We are created in the image of a creative God who looked at creation and felt a sense of pleasure in His work. The Genesis account describes God's joy as He looked at the results of His labor and said, "It is good."

Few experiences in my life are more rewarding than the joy of feeling good about my labors. And yet, when I look at my hammock hanging between the two big pine trees, I want to learn how to use it more effectively. If I felt this to be only a personal dilemma, I would stop at this point. Yet my observations of friends, professional associates, and acquaintances indicate to me a problem of much larger scale.

2

The "Hurry Up and Rest" Syndrome

An old saying that has been passed around in the Army for many years is, "Hurry up and wait." The phrase needs little explanation since we have all found ourselves doing so, whether in the Army or elsewhere. Another phrase more accurately describes my life, "Hurry up and rest." While I have reason to believe most of you understand exactly what I mean, allow me to explain what has become a very frustrating description of my life. The frustration has come from all the hurrying, while seldom getting around to the resting.

The "Hurry Up and Rest" syndrome comes from the belief that, if we hurry enough and get everything in order, we will have a sweet period of resting as a reward for all of our rushing. We willingly pay the price because we anticipate that leisure time when we can relax and have none of these responsibilities hanging over our heads.

These hurry-up periods can be both short term and long term. Allow me to give you a good example of a short-term hurry up. My wife and I both are employed. She teaches in an elementary school, and I am a minister. Therefore, our schedules are rather hectic at times.

Combine our routines with the schedules of our two children and, like most American families, the result is what one psychologist refers to as routine panic. We all covet those occasional evenings when no one has to go anywhere and we can actually sit around the dinner table and introduce ourselves to each other.

Obviously, evenings go better when most of the chores have been done. So, one morning recently I decided to use my lunch hour to get some things done at home so that we would have some leisure time together. I made a determined drive home at lunch and really got busy. I picked up, cleaned up, straightened up, and made up as much as I could. I was proud of my hustle for two reasons. First, how impressed I was with myself for swallowing my masculine pride and doing all of those domestic duties! How impressed my wife would be, and surely my endeavors would be worth a few points and I can normally use all I can get. Second, I was doing all of this hurrying up so that we could rest when everyone came home for the evening.

Within an hour or so I left the house and headed back to the office. I was wet with sweat, hungry, and out of breath. But it was worth all of the effort because we were going to rest that evening.

The evening came. Did the leisurely togetherness occur? If it did, I missed it. I was late getting home. My wife had not bought groceries that week and had to go to the local market. My daughter had a year and a half's worth of homework to do, and my son had a youth meeting that he had forgotten about. All I could think of was, *How profitable and worthwhile was my hurried up lunch hour!* The night was not a total loss. Nights are never bad when we, as a family, are together, even for a short while. But I felt very frustrated because I had done so much rushing around and didn't get to enjoy the dividend I had anticipated. No great tragedy but frustrating none the less!

We periodically have those long-term "hurry up and rest" experiences. Some fall into the category of slight aggravation while others border on the edge of misery. I happen to be writing this chapter with Christmas only two weeks away. One of the goals I set for myself a number of months ago was that I would start preparation early enough that the last few days preceding Christmas would be relaxed and pleasant. I determined in my mind that I wouldn't fall victim to the hysterical panic of Christmas.

Also, I made the industrious decision to make the majority of my Christmas gifts. I thoroughly enjoy woodworking, and the time spent in my shop is usually quite therapeutic. I made a long list of gifts I would build for friends and work associates. I would please them with crafty, eclectic gifts and also impress them with just how talented I am. In order to accomplish such a task, I would start very early and get all of the work finished by Thanksgiving.

My efforts were sincere. On several Saturday mornings I was up at the crack of dawn, busy with my work. I used lunch hours on a couple of days to buy materials in case I had some free evenings I could spend in the shop. The hurrying would be worth the price because I could sit back and enjoy December the way Christmas should be enjoyed.

I am not sure what happened because, at the point of this writing, Christmas is only a few days away and not one of the gifts is finished. Twenty-eight gifts have been

started and within the next week, which contains about a
dozen Christmas parties, I must finish those gifts. My intentions were good. I had hurried as much as possible.
But, even with my honorable goals, frustration was the
result and not the joy of the Christmas season.

Some of the long-term "hurry up and rest" experiences
are considerably more painful. I have opportunities to
share in many of the experiences of people. Frequently I
see these people without their usual facades. If I could
pick one word to describe most of these people, I would
choose the word *tired*. While all kinds of words are thrown
around to describe our society today, such as depressed,
angry, and disillusioned, the word *tired* is more descrip-
tive of the people I know.

Within so many of them the feeling exists that rest is
needed, but they don't know how to go about arranging
such an experience. On a recent Wednesday evening
after our midweek service, one of our church's most active young men came by to visit with me in my study. He
looked very tired and asked if he might have a couple of
minutes. He is an engineer, is extremely intelligent, and
is progressing in his career. He is providing his family all
the nice things that the average family desires. And yet all
over this good man's face was the image of one very close
to burnout.

He described for me the circumstances of why he came
to Augusta. As a veteran in managing complex contruc-
tion projects, he was given the electrical responsibilities
of getting unit one "on line" at a nearby nuclear power
plant. He had spent the past year doing just that and met
the goal. Yet, the price was rather high because the job
required tremendous amounts of time, great amounts of
energy, and a great deal of stress that weighed heavy at
the plant site and at home. Fortunately, he had the sup-

port of his family and friends and survived the demands placed upon him.

One of his sources of motivation was the belief that, by getting the job done, a more restful pace could be assumed. In other words, hurry up and get it done because rest is on the way. Now he finds himself in a dilemma. With unit one nearing completion his immediate supervisor, for whom he has great respect, has requested that he take on unit two. How could he say no to a friend and another challenge? All of the hurrying up and the pressure-filled days of the past year did not bring the rest that was anticipated.

In one way or another we have all been there. At times we can only sit back and laugh at our futile efforts to rest. On other occasions the pain and frustration are very real and intense.

Rest is not a single dynamic. Rest is a discipline that requires thought, planning, and effort. At times we can hurry up and get assignments done and then experience a nice break. At other times, hurrying up to rest doesn't work.

3

Rest, a Cultural Dilemma

A subtle but relatively accurate method of determining the "wants" of our culture is to observe the ways the advertising market appeals to people at any given time. With money as a motivator, the market is a genius at knowing what people want, whether they need it or not. In addition, the market may know what people need whether they want it or not. The appeal of the market through its advertising is a mirror of what our society desires.

From the many suggestions offered by the advertising media, we can assume that rest is an obvious need in our culture. With wisdom to quickly recognize the needs of our life-style and with the speed of modern technology, the market can throw at us more solutions to our problems of unrest than we can digest.

Some of the suggestions are genuine and wise. Others are attempts to take advantage of a culture that is generally exhausted and quite frustrated. A rather quick review of some of the media's recommendations leaves me with two impressions. First, most are superficial. They do not go far enough because they deal primarily with symptoms of the problem of unrest. A new "reclinaway chair" may sit well and match perfectly the decor of the family room but do nothing about a certain life-style that is overcommitted and undermaintained. Another commercial claims that, "It just doesn't get any better than this." However, I would raise a question as to whether the particular moment to which they are referring is essentially rest or escape.

Second, many of the pressures from today's marketing are misleading and take advantage of many people who are desperate for genuine rest. Most of us are so out of touch with our real needs that we fall for advertising gimmicks. We must keep in mind the goal of the market. The market is not motivated by compassion. Determining needs of people and selling products that propose to meet those needs is the name of the game. Buying everything that is held in front of us will not satisfy our deep needs for rest. In fact, thoughtless check writing may have just the opposite effect.

When very little honest attention is given to what we really need, we are subject to every fad that hits the television screen and the Sunday sale paper. We have an obvious need or the market would not offer so many suggestions. The recommendations are varied and endless, and they come at us from all directions.

Recently I had to accept the fact that my son had outgrown his bunk beds. Just because they were mine and served me well until college did not negate the fact that my son was too tall for them. We went to a local furniture store where a salesman met us with answers to our questions before we had time to ask them.

Consistent with my normal tradition, I was interested

in the cheap sets. I did not get much support from the rest
of the family, and the salesman made me feel like a crook.
This man had obviously practiced his monologue many
times. He quickly reminded me that we were talking
about my son's rest and that this was neither the time nor
place to be cheap. I have to give him credit for mention-
ing one fact, that we spend a third of our lives in bed and
a good mattress and springs is a small price to pay for that
amount of time. To be honest I never really thought
before that a man at age seventy-five has spent twenty-
five years in bed, although such a thought is quite pleasant.

The answer to my son's need for rest was an "ultra"
sleep set, guaranteed to bring hours of bliss. This sleep set
was the answer for rest. How could I turn down such an
appeal?

I certainly do not question the virtue of a quality mattress and springs. However, I could not help thinking how
I wish rest were as simple as spending a lot of money on
a bed set. Unfortunately, our rest needs are not so easily
satisfied.

If we recognize that rest is more than sleep, we may
discover another possible solution to our problems of unrest. I occasionally receive invitations in the mail to visit
a new vacation development. In fact, if I go before midnight Friday, I will receive one night's lodging, a free
television, a VCR, three meals, and a chance to win a new
Boeing 747. Doe-Dun-Run is the answer to our struggle
for rest. Nestled in the mountains with tennis courts, golf
course, fishing lake, ski jump, parachute jump, and the
world's next best water slide, these lots will provide the
perfect getaway for today's busy family. For ten thousand
dollars down and ten thousand dollars a month, the Doe-

Dun-Run Corporation will design, finance, and build you the most restful environment known to modern man.

There are a couple of drawbacks to the Doe-Dun-Run concept of rest. If we are honest, most of us do not easily produce the surplus funds for such a project. Regardless of how picturesque the setting might be, the bill must be paid. For some families already under financial stress, the additional demands on their resources compel one to work longer hours to produce the money. Rest can become very expensive!

Another problem comes at the point of the regular visits. You've bought the place, so you must use it. You feel guilty when you don't use it. Trips to this haven of rest are made out of obligation rather than joy. When you go, there are always chores to which attention must be given. Leisure may be the goal but maintenance cannot be ignored. Most getaways require considerable routine upkeep.

Several years ago my family and I purchased a cabin on a large lake. The setting was perfect for rest and retreat. There was a boathouse, a dock, a swimming pool, and a cabin that, naturally, needed a few minor repairs. In the three years that we owned the cabin, I can never remember going without facing some kind of work that needed to be performed. The grass would grow overnight, the swimming pool could turn green while we were eating lunch, a faucet was always leaking, and trash seemed to grow from the flower beds. In three years I never fished once. By the time I got the limbs picked up, the grass cut, and "whatever else" was pressing at the moment, the time of rest was over and it was time to pack up and head back toward home.

I am not taking a "shot" at cabins on the lake and in the mountains. If you enjoy all that is involved in such a project, have at it! But, be careful that you do not set rest as your goal. Some settings are more prone toward rest than others. Condominiums require less maintenance, but the upkeep costs more.

There are many legitimate reasons for investing in beach and mountain getaways. However, you will do yourself a genuine favor by having a clear idea as to why you are making such an investment. When handled carefully one can make some good financial returns on certain properties. Others may choose to purchase a place strictly for the fun and adventure in a certain environment.

However, if rest is your goal, be careful. There are some developments today which provide maintenance support to relieve one of most of the duties relating to upkeep. These services are usually rather expensive, but they do allow the owners to enjoy their getaway with little upkeep responsibility, provided one can afford the assessments.

Most getaways must be maintained by the owners and, if rest is the primary reason for owning such a place, frustration may be the result. For the average family who enjoys getting away once or twice a year for rest and recreation they will come much closer to their goal by renting a "condo" from someone. Pay your money, pick up your keys, enjoy the restful time together, return your keys, and let the owners maintain and repair. Everybody wins. The owners get the return on their investment, and you can relax and rest instead of worrying about any number of repairs that could be made.

The key once again is found in determining your reasons for investing in Doe-Dun-Run Estates. One may have the financial resources and still not choose to make the leap. Even when we seek to provide restful environments for our family we should be careful. In our attempts to promote the comfort of our families the guilt of our own spirit is often disturbed. When overfatigued we cannot contribute to our own pleasure or that of anyone else.

Dr. Julius Johnson, a psychiatrist at University Hospital in Augusta, Georgia, has offered some very practical advice, "If you want to rest, leave home. As long as you are in the house you can usually think of a dozen things to do. Check into a motel where you cannot fix anything or find something that needs to be done." In other words, physical separation from stress agents can usually be a helpful practice.

The first main source of stress for most people is their job. The second main source of stress is the house in which they live. Some people may discover that unless they can periodically get away from both they will never relax. A house for most of us is much more than just shelter. A house becomes one's sense of territory. It frequently becomes an extension of our personality, and we use the house we live in to gain status and approval from our peers. We frequently go to great extremes to produce a house that will enhance our community position.

The stress comes from overextending ourselves financially and by our compulsive need for perfection in appearance. When we are at home we notice a dozen things that could be done immediately. A compulsive personality may particularly experience a problem at this point since he can settle for very little less than perfection.

Anyone who has owned a home for more than an hour knows that perfection is an illusive dream. While homeowning may be the American dream, it can also be one of the most serious sources of unrest in our society. Houses require continual maintenance. Unless one learns how to handle the inevitable demands of homeowning, a house can become a nightmare.

A pleasant and healthy experience of homeowning can be attributed to at least three factors. First, one must have a realistic attitude about what a house really is. A house is, first and foremost, shelter. Yes, it can be pretty, comfortable, and even spacious. But when a house becomes too closely tied to our personalities, we are in for trouble.

Second, one must make upkeep and maintenance a regular activity; not continuous, just regular. A little bit of discipline goes a long way. To do a little along the way is much better than letting it build up to an overwhelming task. Very little sympathy can be offered to one who cannot relax in his or her house because it is so dirty and yet the last serious housecleaning took place before grandmother's funeral twelve years ago.

Third, one must learn how to rest and relax in a house that is not perfect. Few attain the perfect dwelling place. Even the wealthy who can afford their domestic desires can always become preoccupied in the next addition or the next edition. There is always something that could be done.

There is another advertisement that intrigues me. "Come home each evening and relax around your pool. Provide yourself with the perfect setting for rest." Let's be honest, pools are fun and can be a lovely addition to one's home, but we should be careful not to equate them with rest. I am not on a campaign against pools. I have owned one and am considering building another, but not for rest. The point is that once again we must be honest about our intention and not mislead ourselves. Pools may be fun and pretty, but they also require work.

We had one that could turn green in a matter of minutes. There was always a repair that needed to be done. I once spent weeks trying to find a leak in the liner. While we were away for a week the water leaked out—that's right, the whole pool. Where can that much water go? I accused my neighbor of irrigating his flowers and lawn out of my pool. He thought I was teasing. I was serious. Finally we found the crack, replaced the liner, and were able to keep water in the pool.

There are moments of relaxation by the pool. However, those moments do not come without work. I now pay a fee to a neighborhood pool and let them vacuum and scrub. When I have finished swimming, I can return home and let someone else keep the water from turning green.

The point is very simple. As with other things, be honest about your intentions. If you want a pool because of its beauty, capacity for fun, or opportunities for exercise, go after it. If you want a pool because a dealer told you that it was the ideal environment for rest, go straight home and lock yourself in the house until you come to your senses.

On and on we could go with all kinds of suggestions from the market about how to solve our problems of unrest. Most attempts rarely get below the surface. The issue of rest is too personal to be dealt with in wholesale fashion. The secret of not being misled is just a little bit of honesty.

In our society there truly must exist a general state of fatigue. Otherwise, why the appeal from the market in a thousand ways? Too many of us can relate to this experience of a couple who are friends of mine. They were watching television one night and both were having some difficulty staying awake. Midway through their favorite program Ann was standing up as she watched. When questioned why, she replied, "The only way I can stay awake and see how it ends is to stand up." We have all been there!

Rest will not come from purchasing chairs and beach houses and swimming pools. Rest will come when we maintain a disciplined mind, a healthy emotional state, a controlled physical body, and an effective spiritual life to undergird and overarch one's life. Leave any one of these dimensions out and we will be subject to every gimmick we see and hear.

The point I am trying to make is very simple. If the market is an indicator of our personal desires as a society, there must be an obvious need for rest. On the other hand, we cannot depend totally on the market because its motivation is to sell a product and not necessarily to create a more restful society. We must take responsibility for ourselves.

4

A Definition of Rest

If we are to move toward a more effective process of rest, we must have a more clearly defined description of this activity. To describe rest as an activity may seem contradictory, particularly if we have understood rest to be an absence of activity. On the contrary, rest should not be understood in such passive terms.

Instead of rest being the result of not doing anything, meaningful rest occurs as a result of something that is done. Rest is not a state of passivity, but, rather, the involvement of one's total self in a creative process. Rest might be better understood as a discipline.

Several facts must be acknowledged at this point in this new approach of rest. First, such an understanding of rest appears, on the surface, to be paradoxical to the normal definition of rest. Webster defines rest as, "The act or state of ceasing from work, activity, or motion." This approach to rest is entirely too passive. The implication is that cessation from motion or activity is all that is needed for rest to occur. Most of us can think of nights when activity had ceased but rest was far from reality.

Second, rest is an intentional endeavor of one's self. Instead of withdrawing, one deliberately involves mind, body, and soul in a discipline that becomes a creative process. A comparison might be made with the conceptual change a few years ago in the understanding of listening. Instead of listening being a passive activity, it began to be understood as an art and, even more specifically, as something done actively. Effective listening involves more than just passively receiving sounds.

John Drakeford wrote a significant book in 1967 entitled *The Awesome Power of the Listening Ear*. Drakeford's basic premise was that listening is an art in which people actively engage. There is the physiological process of listening and then there is the active art of listening. In a similar way, rest must be understood as more than the absence of "hustle and bustle" of everyday existence.

A fourth fact must be acknowledged. Rest must not be used interchangeably with such words as *relaxation* and *recreation*. While each of these processes bear some similarities, they are at best cousins, not brothers and sisters. Relaxation is both mental and physical but is usually understood as the lessening of physical tension, particularly in regard to muscles. Recreation is also a positive activity and is usually understood as the refreshment of mind and body. One can participate in recreation, enjoy it, but be worn-out when it is done. Rest, however, involves all these processes and more.

Rest occurs on a deeper level than relaxation or recreation. Relaxation and recreation can take us only so far. Rest becomes the vehicle for translating tired and confused people into energetic people with hope and dignity and the desire to once again be creative. Conceivably, criticism might be offered that this approach to rest is taking something that should be simple and making something complex out of it. Without a doubt, the world is complicated enough! Are we making a "mountain out of a mole hill"? The goal is definitely not to make life more complicated. The goal is to increase the effectiveness of our rest. In fact, striving toward simplicity is precisely one of those ways in which we bring about a more adequate routine of rest.

At the risk of redundancy, one point will be stated again and again in this book and must be clearly understood if rest is to have any value at all: Rest cannot and must not be perceived as only the absence of physical activity. This one fact is precisely the point of confusion for many people who find themselves continually in a state of exhaustion.

Dr. Wayne Hodges of the Savannah Pain Clinic, in an interview concerning rest, offered a very practical example of rest being more than inactivity. Such a premise can be demonstrated by patients who have come to him and allowed themselves to be placed on bio-feedback. In an interview he said, "In taking them [patients] through some Jacobsonean procedures of deep muscle relaxation, some have commented that they do this kind of thing all the time at home through yoga or meditation, or some other technique they learned from television late one night. Some of these patients might demonstrate how well they can relax and from all appearances they have are truly resting." Then, however, Dr. Hodges attached electrodes to the patients and measured the microvoltage level of their muscles. This procedure is an indirect way of measuring the autonomic nervous system input to those muscles which indicates the level of tension. The findings were totally different from what the patients had verbalized. The microvoltage indicated anything but a state of rest.

Dr. Hodges said, "Even a physician learns quickly that one's overt appearance has little to do with what is going on under the skin. The most intriguing thing about the process is that patients will say that they are relaxed, but their physiological arousal level is anything but relaxed. That is particularly so with many persons who suffer from tension headaches." He added, "I treat many people with migraine, tension, and scalp muscle contracture headaches who believe that they are relaxed. They have bought book after book and watched programs on television and think they have it all down pat. But, they do not."

In spite of what your favorite dictionary might offer, rest is more than a period of refraining from physical activity. Inactivity is an important part of the process, but rest that is effective involves much more. It is the response of the total person to the demands of living; this response must incorporate one's physical, mental, emotional, and spiritual capacities. Rest should also be seen as the process of preparing for those demands which are to follow. In other words, rest is not the end of the game. It is a temporary time-out for the purpose of getting back into the game.

There is risk involved whenever we try to divide ourselves into nice, neat categories. To say that effective rest involves our physical, mental, emotional, and spiritual capacities runs such a risk of over simplification. Personality cannot be that easily divided. At any one time, more than one capacity is always operational. The division is made only for clarification and understanding.

Rest is not an end, but is a means to an end. Rest is the process by which one intentionally and actively experiences the revitalizing and refreshing processes made available by our Creator. To consider such a process as a discipline is not to make a "mountain out of a molehill," rather it gives rest the place in our lives that it deserves.

5

Rest and the Human Body

From a physiological perspective, what purpose does rest serve? Dr. Charles Shaefer, a private-practice internist, concisely described rest as, "nature's way of providing that period of readjustment that is necessary in order to properly interact with one's environment." Such a definition can be easily observed in the animal kingdom. Consider, for example, the annual routine of the bears which hibernate in the winter. During a time when their food is difficult to find, they enter into this very restful, inactive state of almost suspended animation. As a result, they are able to interact with their environment in an efficient and favorable way.

While we don't practice hibernation, human beings depend upon rest for the same purpose, that is to interact efficiently and favorably with our environment. If we are to develop more effective habits of rest in our life-styles, we need to have a better understanding of what takes place within our bodies physiologically. Such a consideration might initially appear somewhat elementary. Yet, if we were honest, most of us would admit that we know very little about the processes of the human body. While my basic thrust in these pages has been that rest involves much more than the physiological, certainly the physical dimension must not be omitted from our understanding. As we become more informed concerning our bodies, we can be more sensitive to the healthy and unhealthy ways we are responding to our environment. Remember, also, that our bodies will frequently give us advance signals about potential breakdowns if we are sensitive and informed enough to take note of what is going on within us. Unfortunately the fact is that most of us pay little attention to the messages that come from our bodies. Consider the man who is working two jobs, restoring an old house, coaching his son's soccer team, and always has a cold and becomes personally acquainted with every new virus that passes through the county. If he were to notice the plea that his body is making, he might make some adjustments in his life-style and avoid a more serious and inevitable breakdown.

In preparation for this book I was somewhat surprised as I began to survey the available scientific research on rest. In spite of the fact that rest was a part of God's original plan, the field is relatively new and wide open as a general area of study. Most of what we know about rest comes as a spin-off from other related research efforts, such as sleep disorders, stress, muscular relaxation, and many other specific areas which have received attention in past years. No one, to my knowledge, has tried to relate them under one general field of research and develop the concept of rest as a discipline. Such a field of study seems desparately needed in our tired and overcommitted society.

Never doubt that without adequate rest our body will

eventually break down. While some people are constitu-
tionally stronger than others and, therefore, can function
under great stress longer than others, sooner or later
physiological problems will occur. Consider one of the old
schools of psychology called constitutional psychology.
This particular school of thought was formulated on the
idea that the body has a hierarchy of organ systems that
respond to stress.

According to the theories of constitutional psychology,
stress levels are expressed differently among persons so
that in a normal day of activity the most vulnerable system will vary from one person to another. For one person
it might be the heart. For another person it might be the
lung system or the gastrointestinal tract or some other
bodily system. When one's health fails (when one
becomes ill), the breakdown is a result of, at least, one
system which failed. All things being equal, the system
that fails will be the one that is weakest in the chain;
unless there is a reversal, the next system to fail will be the
next weakest. Our bodily systems work like a chain; when
placed under enough discomfort, the weakest link in the
chain will break. This theory is true only for nonorganic
or pathologic diseases. In other words, much depends on
the nature of the invading organism which could be the
source of the stress.

Many of us operate with a relatively limited understanding of our body and how our body responds to the
great demands placed upon it. Most of us have certain
problems that occur when we are subjected to stress. In
fact, certain symptoms may become barometers of our
stress level, and that is not necessarily all bad. We need to
be conscious of our bodies. If we are familiar with our own
physiological constitution, we can learn to read our bodies

in such a way so as to become aware of increased stress levels.

You might have heard someone say that we are all wired differently in the way we respond to stress. When under stress, some people develop headaches. For others, intestinal problems can be expected. For others heart problems become apparent. These different responses do mean that, physiologically, the nerves of some persons are necessarily wired to their organs differently than in other people. From one person to another a stress response is very similar. The breakdowns of a certain organ results from that organ being the weakest in the chain.

The fact that a certain person responds to periods of great demand with intestinal problems does not necessarily mean that a serious illness is imminent in that system of the body. That particular system's breakdown occurs because in comparison with one's other systems the problematic area simply is the weakest in the chain. Organ systems tend to fail in a hierarchical manner according to which one is weakest and will correspond to the physical constitution of a given individual. One's "wires" are not hooked up to a certain organ as much as that particular organ is the weakest and stress causes the problem to surface. The particular organ is not necessarily inferior in its ability to function. Instead, the problem is the first signal that one is overstressed. If we are wise, we will become familiar with our own uniqueness and learn to read our bodies which have an amazing ability to signal us that we are not getting adequate rest or that we are not dealing with stress in a very healthy manner.

The body may respond in a variety of ways to long periods of stress and, more specifically, to the abuse of poor rest habits. While some persons have a physical constitution that is stronger than others, no one can indefi-

nitely ignore the need of adequate rest. Sooner or later a
physiological breakdown will occur.

Based upon the work of Dr. Hans Selye and other physicians who have studied the physiological response to
stress, we now know that much of the immune system is
involved in the stress response. An example to which most
of us can relate is the tendency to get a cold during a
period of stress or after a long period of physical exertion.

The immune system of the body can be viewed as an
army of small soldiers of cells that are able to conduct
physical combat and chemical warfare. Dr. Wayne
Hodges of the Savannah Pain Clinic in Savannah, Georgia,
has described the immune system as, "An army of cells
which actually smother and take hold of harmful organisms which enter the body system. They are capable of
literally squirting chemicals that kill organisms and com-
municate to other body organs to make certain defenses
against disease and illness."

During long periods of stress and unrest, the body's
immune system becomes impaired or, at least, compro-
mised. The exact reasons are rather technical but are
primarily a result of increased levels of catecholamines
which begin to impair the response of the immune system. The important thing for us to know is that frequently
illness is brought on as a direct result of poor rest habits
and long periods of stress. One who rests well will usually
do better at resisting some types of illnesses.

Most of us can recall a time when we were dealing with
some rather intense demands. The long-term stress and
chronic fatigue resulted in a bad cold, as well as some
strong feelings of depression. Our assumption is that colds
usually come from physical overexposure, which is not the
case according to recent research. Experimental research
has found that exposure to extreme cold does not lead to

colds. Colds are passed primarily by hand-to-mouth contact. Hand-to-mouth contact between persons occur more
often during the cold months when people are inside
more and are in closer contact. Yet, lack of rest compro-
mises the immune response which means higher risk of
acquiring a cold when exposed to the virus. No physician
would deny that colds are enhanced by subjecting the
body to unhealthy temperatures or that we catch colds
from each other. What we fail to realize is that the most
important factor in the whole process is the body's immune system.

I can think of one particular psychiatrist who has taken
the extreme position that colds come not from physical
overexposure but emotional overexposure and the related stress response of the body. While the position of the
psychiatrist may be a bit extreme for most of us, the point
is well made.

The immune system does become impaired during
periods of stress. That is why we fall victim to many infec-
tions during times of great demands. So much is yet to be
learned and discovered in this field of study. If we knew
more, we could even correct the problems of the common
cold. Few physicians would debate the fact that adequate
rest (and washing your hands) is a good defense against
the common cold.

As a result of recent discoveries about the relationship
of the immune system to stress and fatigue, a new field of
medicine is developing called Neuro-Psycho Immunolo-
gy. The whole idea behind this perspective is that one's
emotional state affects the immune system vastly and that
changes can be made which increase the body's resistance
to infection.

Much of what happens to our bodies during the cycle
of work-rest is quite obvious and requires no great techni-

cal understanding. One half of the cycle is the body's labor process and the other half is the process of restoring cells to equilibrium. The labor process involves the consumption of energy, including the production of waste products; and the restoration process involves the replenishing of energy in the cells. The restoration process is absolutely necessary if the cells are to continue to function. The Crebbs Johnson Lactic Acid Cycle is the process by which the energy in a muscle cell is replenished. The cycle is a very intriguing process of efficiency within the body. One physician has compared the cycle within the muscle to the firing of an automobile engine. Glucose and oxygen come together in the muscle like gasoline and air in a carburetor. The glucose and oxygen then produce ATP molecules which become the source of energy for the muscle. When finely tuned, however, the body is much more efficient. Waste products such as lactic acid are converted into the sequence and the cycle eventually begins again. The cycle is very necessary as a response to the physical activity of the muscle and the breakdown of energy-producing products.

The bottom line is that, regardless of how strong one considers himself or herself to be, muscular activity cannot go on forever without rest. Otherwise, lactic acid and other waste products will accumulate to the point that a muscle cannot contract at all. While effective rest involves much more than just physical inactivity, periods of muscular relaxation are certainly a vital part of the process. From a physiological process rest cannot be ignored.

One area in which our society is being misled today is in regard to chemicals that supposedly enhance the work-rest cycle. Many of the chemicals we assume to be helpful essentially interfere with the cycle. Some chemicals are purchased as drugs while others are a part of our diet.

Once the work-rest cycle is interrupted, one frequently has difficulty in establishing the natural rhythm again.

The subject of sleep has been given considerable attention in recent days, even more specifically the study of sleep disorders. While there has been an intensified effort in the past few years to study this area, most physicians will admit that they just do not understand much about it. Most of the medical attention has been given to the physiology of sleep and continues to be a subject of significant interest and research.

Sleep is an undeniably vital part of the resting process. Sleep occurs through various stages, cycling through a very superficial sleep and dropping into a very deep sleep. Sleep may be defined quite simply as a cessation of the routine, purposeful physical and mental activities. We have learned that all sleep is not the same. In fact, one might go as far as to distinguish useful sleep and nonuseful sleep. The useful sleep is the REM (rapid eye movement) sleep that we drop into periodically throughout the night. We cycle through these periods of REM sleep which usually last from thirty to ninety minutes.

Most of the REM sleep occurs in the early morning hours. Such a theory might provide justification for those who like to sleep late and use as an excuse that one might be subject to more REM sleep. The stage tends to occur at the end of the cycle and provides the quality sleep which gives the revitalization that people need.

Recent research into sleep disorders can explain why some people do not sleep well. They may sleep for rather long periods of time but wake up feeling very tired. After analyzing their situation they may find that a drug or some other problem is inhibiting the REM sleep. For example, too much alcohol will interfere with REM sleep.

One may be sleeping for eight hours but the quality stage of sleep just is not there.

Sleep is necessary for revitalization, and the lack of sleep can also become a significant source of anxiety. Many feel that the only restful sleep is a deep sleep where one is really out of it. For those who have difficulty in sleep and those who are not satisfied with their sleep pattern, the temptation is to resort to chemically induced sleep. There are times when artificially induced sleep is necessary but should be done very carefully.

The frustrating dimension of chemically induced sleep is that it frequently does not provide the quality recuperation of natural sleep. There is considerable difference between the rehabilitative capacities of natural sleep and chemically induced sleep. Most of the cell-replenishing ability of sleep comes during REM sleep. For some reason REM does not occur as readily in chemically induced sleep. The drug interferes with the process. The result is that frequently one who is taking sleeping pills will be sleeping more and more and yet feeling increasingly worse and cannot understand why.

One of the big-selling features of several drugs is that they supposedly do not interfere with REM sleep. However, very few sleep-inducing drugs, if any, do not interfere with sleeping patterns. One physician has described a very typical pattern of a person who depends on a particular drug for sleep. The patient is initially satisfied with the results of the drug. His eyes have been closed, and he slept for eight hours. He should feel good but, quite honestly, he feels lousy. After a few days or weeks the patient will call the doctor again and say that the medication isn't working and another one is then tried. All of these drugs are basically desensitizing the recepter mechanisms of the brain so that the patient is becoming less and less sensitive to the hypnotic effect of the medication.

The point is that one needs REM sleep. This is the quality sleep and everything else is "window dressing." REM sleep rests tired muscles, soothes aching joints, and revitalizes the system. Dr. Charles Shaefer said, "The stuff of sleep that makes you capable of functioning intellectually, emotionally, spiritually, and physically is REM sleep. It is what enables you to adapt to the stresses of the environment."

The active side of the work-rest cycle is also influenced. The body cannot always cooperate with the timetable of our schedule. We must "get up and get with it," but our bodies are still under the influence of the chemical. Therefore, we resort to another chemical to offset our sluggishness. The most common chemical to pick us up is caffeine. This stimulant creates a chemical process which extracts a "price" from our system, creating a demand upon a system that is already tired.

The body, through the pineal gland, has its own time-clock and all our downers and uppers constantly work against the natural rhythm of the body and more specifically the work-rest cycle. At times of stress, illness, or injury, we may need substances to support and enhance the rhythm of the body. However, if at the first sign of restlessness one goes to the medicine cabinet, the symptoms have become the focus not the underlying problems. The real issues are frequently masked by our quick dependency upon drugs.

Rest is essential for us. We cannot ignore the needs of our bodies to restore and replenish that which was lost due to activity. The natural rhythm demanded by our body is an intriguing process. Our productivity as human beings depends upon a following through of the cycle. Ignore the need and breakdown is inevitable.

When rest is denied, the functioning of the body is directly affected. There is a gradual diminishing of abilities all the way down the biogenetic scale. There is first a lessening of intellectual sharpness. The process can continue all the way to the basic bodily functions involving brain stem failure which determines respiration, blood pressure, and pulse. The ultimate extreme would be death if the process were not reversed.

The lesson we can learn at this point is quite obvious. Poor rest habits negatively affect our functioning. While few people have ever gone to the extreme of death by exhaustion, many of us have experienced the upper end of the scale when our mental abilities have been reduced due to fatigue. One of the first indicators of fatigue is a lessening of intellectual sharpness. Our recall capacity is diminished. We may not be able to respond as quickly as we normally would. The process could continue to a state of confusion.

Adequate rest, particularly through sleep, is not optional. Sleep is a necessary part of the natural rhythm and while the amount of sleep needed varies with the individual, sleep is a right one must claim.

The average person needs seven to eight hours of sleep but that time can be reduced with training. The number of hours of sleep needed is genetically determined. One particular surgeon trained himself to function on one hour of sleep per night. This man is one of a very few people who has the right combination of native stamina and sleep patterns. He is the exception, not the rule.

Most medical students can attest to both the need and training aspects of sleep. Interns and residents are frequently subjected to long hours of responsibility with little time for sleep. Most medical students learn to get by on less sleep and train themselves to make better use of the opportunities for sleep. On the other hand, they can also describe many agonizing experiences of trying to make critical decisions under the influence of fatigue.

Studies have been done with medical residents in regard to sleep deprivation. One such study included in the *Annals of Internal Medicine* in 1987 dealt with the effect of sleep loss on residents having to stay awake for long periods of time. Interestingly, for those forced to stay awake, the blood pressure tended to be higher, pulse rate faster, and rapid mental recall became slower when compared to a control group with similar circumstances except for the loss of sleep.

Just as one inherits a certain degree of physical strength, there is also the natural granting of certain sleep patterns. Sleep patterns also change. Older persons may need less sleep. Eight hours sleep per day may not be necessary for everyone. In fact, the quest for sleep can become an inhibiting factor. There is a feeling with some persons that one absolutely must have eight hours of sleep or "the wheels will fall off." Anxiety about sleep can create enough tension to actually prohibit sleep. One must take care to envision sleep as a right and not as a forced obligation. Since one third of our lives is spent sleeping, we would do well to learn more about the process of sleep. Yet most of us are quite ignorant about what actually transpires during that time.

One current concern of medical science is in the area of what actually happens to the body during sleep. There are many unanswered questions that need attention. For example, we know that the majority of a child's growth actually occurs during the sleeping hours. It is also believed that a child's bones get longer during sleep. This is the time when much of our physiological growth takes place.

There is another dimension of our bodies about which we should be aware. Consider the vital role our glandular system plays in our work and in our rest. The pituitary gland is a master gland that directs the hormonal activity of the whole body. Located near the pituitary is the very intriguing pineal gland. For a long time this gland has gone relatively unnoticed, but now medical science has begun to realize that in animals this gland tells them when to hibernate, when to get up, and determines much of their work-rest cycle.

A group of French scientists decided to test the influence of the pineal gland in the human body. They locked themselves in caves for long periods of time and tried drastically to disorient themselves. They made notes about whether it was day or night and when the days would begin and end. The results at the end of these experiments were remarkably accurate in measuring twenty-four hour days. Something "inside" of them seemed to tell them that twenty-four hours had passed or, in other words, one complete day-night cycle. Interestingly, they maintained cycles of wakefulness and sleeping with no distractions and totally devoid of external stimuli. They were still able to function on relatively accurate cycles of sleep and rest. Medical science is pointing to the pineal gland as a master clock operating within our body.

The pineal is able to convey messages to other organs in the body. Time cycling, such as day-night or work-rest cycling, is a key element in the entire organism. Much of our hormonal activity functions in a cyclical fashion. Therefore, our waking and resting is tuned to hormonal behavior. For example, most of us have surges of adrenal hormone in the morning and another during late after-noon. Quite possibly this is a result of the pineal gland, the master clock.

One unfortunate characteristic of our modern culture is that we have become so unaware of the cyclical nature of life. Many people live in such an artificial environment that day and night makes little difference. The seasons come and go and people hardly notice. In an agricultural environment one becomes very close to the earth. The daily cycle and the seasonal cycle provide a base for time as well as a sense of orientation.

Now we live in total-comfort homes with electronically controlled temperatures. With enough concrete, steel, and artificial lighting, day and night means very little. Our generation has suffered a significant loss by moving away from the natural rythmns of life.

The bottom line is that the human body is a masterfully tuned organism. In order to function at its best, adequate rest is a necessity. Our bodies will frequently "tell" us that we are not providing adequate opportunities for rest. These messages may be subtle at first and quite dramatic if allowed to go unnoticed.

While many of us have never suffered from a complete collapse, we do operate at less than peak efficiency. Our lack of mental sharpness and intellectual clarity may very well be a result of inadequate rest.

The next time you cannot remember your spouse's name when making an introduction at a dinner party may be the clue that you are just plain tired. With the realization that one is just plain tired, one might want to take a serious inventory of a life-style that is poorly balanced.

You might also be questioning why you have spent this

time reading something you already know, that adequate rest is necessary for functioning at our best. On the other hand, if this fact is so obvious, why do most of us spend so much time in a state of fatigue?

6

The Avoidance of Ourselves

The year 1984 was a rather difficult one for me and my family. The difficulties came both directly and indirectly for me from two rather serious accidents which occurred within three months of each other. The first was a serious burn from an automobile radiator. The second involved multiple injuries from a motorcycle accident. One year like that is enough for anyone!

In retrospect, I now see those experiences as valuable opportunities for personal growth and, even more importantly, an opportunity to become aware of the workings of God in my life. Just to set the record straight, let me state one opinion from the very beginning. I do not believe God caused the radiator to explode or called for a truck to slam into my son and me while we were riding a motorcycle. Both experiences were a result of my own ineptness and carelessness.

We should be very cautious about ascribing all of our personal dilemmas to God, as though He were a sick parent who finds pleasure in the suffering of His children.

God does maintain control of all of life. He can radically change our circumstances or do away with the entire human experiment with a passing thought if He should choose to do so. Along with His divine power, however, is the element of human freedom which is lovingly granted to us who are created in His image. Some of our sufferings are brought about by our misuse of that freedom. Needless to say, we do experience some hardships which are totally unrelated to our actions, but we do influence much that comes our way. Yet, in all of our circumstances God is at work for good. Every moment and every experience can be placed within His grace, and good can result.

To envision life in such a way has been a challenge for me throughout all my days, and more specifically during the struggles of 1984. I believe very strongly that God used those experiences to teach me some valuable truths about faith and some timely lessons about myself.

I learned, as have others in similar circumstances, that in difficult times God can always be depended upon. Unfortunately many of us must come to our weakest moments before we grasp the strength available to us through the presence of God in our lives. How wise we would be if we could learn that lesson without first having our own strength stripped away. And strength and health can be yanked away with the speed of light!

Now, what does all of this have to do with the issue of rest? These experiences had a profound influence on my understanding of rest. For the purpose of this chapter, I would like to focus attention on one particular dynamic. These accidents, particularly during the recuperation time, forced me to deal with someone whom I have usually done my best to avoid—myself.

The events and subsequent emotions following the motorcycle accident will always be stamped in my memory.

The first few hours were primarily a time of great anxiety for me over the condition of my son. I had some difficulty dealing with the tenuous condition of my own body out of my anxiety that my son was not really OK. I thought the doctors were lying to me. After seeing him with my own eyes and realizing that except for some bruises and scrapes he was going to be OK, I could begin to deal with the issue of life and death for myself. There were some very questionable moments in my mind during those early hours. Soon I sensed that I had avoided death and thought that the struggles were over. The truth is that many of the struggles had just begun.

One of the biggest struggles came during the days of recovery and recuperation. The struggle was primarily in the fact that I was forced to be still and rest. Even with all the manufactured distractions, I had long hours to deal with myself. Plenty of visitors helped to distract me, but, out of courtesy, their visits were brief. After all, my doctor had ordered plenty of rest.

My solitude came by force, not by choice. In spite of a number of broken bones, I had difficulty sitting still. An accident can bring about some immediate changes in one's body, but a life-style just cannot be altered so quickly. My life had always been characterized by activity. Patient waiting was never my long suit. I cannot claim to have accomplished that much, but I have certainly kept the dust stirred up in my attempts. A hurried-up life-style has been my way of approaching life.

For example, I can clearly remember the final days of high school. Most kids will allow some time for fun and rest before entering the college classroom. I felt like I needed to hurry up and begin my college career. And there was a good reason. You must understand a personal secret, and be kind to me by not laughing. By the end of high school I was already losing my hair. Such a problem meant that I needed to hurry up with marriage plans since no young lady would be interested in a bald head. The message from my elders was also clear that marriage should always follow college. So, I had to hurry up with college in order to find a wife before I became bald. I had no lady in mind, but that was beside the point.

Therefore, I graduated from high school on a Friday night and left home for college summer school within three days. And the race was on. From the beginning of my college days, I also knew that post-graduate school must follow. If all of that had to be done, I had to get with the program! There was no other option but to turn on the jets. I finished college in three years.

I graduated from college in summer school and began post-graduate study within a couple of weeks. Most folk have enough sense to take their time and enjoy what is probably the most exciting time of a person's life. I enjoyed the experience but with the usual hurried-up approach.

Seminary went by like a flash. While everything was in place, I felt I would be foolish not to begin doctoral studies. I saw little advantage in moving a wife and child back to the campus later. (By the way, I was able to marry before losing all my hair.) So I began doctoral work and continued with my normal approach to living.

Since that time very little has changed. The setting periodically has changed, but my habits remained strong and thorough. We are creatures of habit and deeply ingrained habits are tough to alter. One can always justify being out of breath when the pace is for honorable causes.

Incidently, I think we frequently encourage such a lifestyle in our local churches. When we think of faithful dedication, the person who usually comes to our mind is the one who is out of breath, attends every meeting, and has no time for the temptations of the world. If one wants to avoid a contemplative life-style, one possible way to do so is to join a local church and attend every function. If it is true that a church leader's prayer concerning the preacher is, "Lord, you keep him humble and we'll keep him poor," then the prayer of a preacher concerning the church leader is, "Lord, you keep him dedicated, and I'll keep him tired." Being out of breath is an effective defense mechanism, for a while.

In 1984 I learned that broken bones listen to no arguments. The body takes charge and, with or without a doctor's order, says, "You are going to sit still for a while." If you think I am making a bigger deal out of this than it deserves, ask some others who have faced such a challenge. Ask any compulsive soul who gets his or her strokes from being overcommitted and out of breath and you will hear a similar story.

Sitting still didn't come easy at first. Pain helped but, fortunately, didn't last forever. Rest is necessary if one is to make a reentry into the world, but rest isn't always easy. Those days of recuperation became a real life laboratory for me, and I had to learn to feel comfortable with myself.

I soon learned to enjoy silence and take advantage of the time to face up to some important issues in my life. I began to consider the meaning of life and death and the meaning of my own existence. I certainly didn't come up with all the answers to the questions in my mind, but I did discover some.

Such a circumstance forced me to deal with my own mortality. Intellectually I knew that my days are numbered, but I had never really accepted such a fact on a practical level. One simply cannot come that close to death and not realize how very thin the line is between life and death.

David once said to his friend Jonathan, "There is but a step between me and death" (1 Sam. 20:3). The majority of us never take such a consideration to heart. We will deny our mortality as long as we can. To deal honestly with ourselves is to claim the fact that we are mortal and someday we are going to die. A look in the mirror underscores the inevitable and irreversible marching of time.

One of the most important lessons I learned is that rest can never become meaningful when one can find no peace within oneself. Avoiding oneself is a very expensive endeavor that causes rest to remain a stranger. A tremendous amount of energy is required to insulate one from oneself. Endless activity will frequently become the means of such an avoidance.

The appearance of fatigue can also become a defense mechanism in relating to other people. I have known people, frequently in service professions, who tell me how tired they are. They even maintain their appearance in such a way as to say, "Don't make any demands of me. I have all I can handle." Fatigue may really be an issue, but the chances are good that such a person simply wants to avoid people. A fatigued appearance is a rather effective way of maintaining distance.

I once worked with a man who, after only a few minutes in his office, would ruffle his hair, unbutton his collar, and loosen his tie. He would sigh and blow as though too much was being demanded of him. One could not help feeling terribly guilty for making a request of him. I never could figure out exactly what he did with his time, so his defense mechanism evidently worked quite well.

Avoiding oneself requires considerably more energy than avoiding others. We get a few breaks along the way when we are trying to maintain distance from other people. Avoiding ourselves is like running from a shadow. We cannot get away from it.

The pattern is very familiar. If I construct enough activity, demands, and routine rush, I indefinitely postpone the scary process of honestly dealing with myself. If I look in the mirror, who will I really see? What will I discover about myself? Will I really meet the phony that I think I am? If who I appear to be is phony, who is the real me? What would I do if I do not like the real me? Is there value to be found in me other than in what I can produce? What would I do if I discovered that I really am the failure I have secretly thought myself to be? These questions and many more come from within as we begin to take an honest look at ourselves.

Most of us would rather not deal with such honest questions about ourselves, and the result is a life in the fast lane which we hope will protect us from such honesty. We may become quite efficient in our defenses until some external circumstance strips our defenses away. We are then left with the task of facing our second best friend, ourselves.

Gerhard Fergsteegan wrote in the seventeenth century:

> Within! within, oh turn
> My spirit's eyes, and learn
> Thy wandering senses gently to control;
> Thy dearest Friend dwells deep within thy soul,
>   and asks thyself of thee,
> That heart, and mind, and sense, He may make whole
>   In perfect harmony.

As a minister I have visited many people in the hospital. There have been numerous times when the patient's biggest problem at the moment was not the condition for which he was admitted. His biggest problem was that he was in a hospital bed with very little to insulate him from the most threatening person in his life—himself. Where can you run when your biggest threat takes every step with you?

To come face to face with ourselves is not always to like what we see. In fact, an honest look may be a bit disquieting. But how can we ever systematically improve our condition unless we first begin as we are? One cannot begin over there; right here is the place.

On the other hand we may discover that we are not as bad as we thought. Our preconceived notions may be misconceptions. Such is the risk we run. The fears we have of ourselves may go back a long way. They may come from early experiences with parents and friends. They may come from vain wanderings of our imaginations. We usually discover that our worst fears are unfounded. We are not nearly as unlovable as we once feared. We discover that we do not have to pretend to be someone else. We can just be ourselves.

How much energy we spend trying to avoid the one person we need most to know! Possibly you are dissatisfied with the closeness of relationships. Quite possibly other people are having trouble getting to know you because you are having precisely the same difficulty with yourself.

Is it not true that many of us spend most of our days wishing we were someone else living in another time and in another place? Joy becomes illusive as long as we are not willing to accept the person we were meant to be. We do not have to even be satisfied with ourselves. One fact is obvious, we cannot grow unless we begin where we are.

Two years after my accident a colleague of mine was injured in an automobile accident. Bob Blankenship, of Harlem, Georgia, suffered severe injuries which forced him to be still for months. On several occasions we talked about the experience and, within appropriate limits, compared notes. Bob also went through the trauma of dealing with his own humanity. I like the way he referred to his experience. Bob called it his "disease," a time when he was both afforded and forced to face up to several areas of who he was as a person.

As he related to me, one of the big issues for him was that of self-identity. Does identity come from being or doing? A very appropriate issue when doing is, for the moment, not an option. "Was I Bob because I was involved in much doing? Was I Bob because I was being a person? Though life is bound up in being and doing, the truth I kept discovering was that Bob was Bob more for being than for doing."

Fortunately one does not have to experience a serious personal injury in order to become at peace with oneself. The real question seems to be whether we can accept the honesty of such an endeavor. To be honest with ourselves means that we must attempt to see ourselves as we really are. What are some possible discoveries? Although everyone's experience is unique, let me suggest some possibilities.

Anger may be a discovery. Anger is a natural emotion, but most of us are not very adept at dealing with it. We often deny it and ignore it. Then we wonder why we made a particular statement that was so out of character and so inappropriate.

Anger is a natural response to an imperfect world. Sometime long ago we may have been told that good people don't get angry. However, even the best people become angry. Good people just know how to direct their emotions into appropriate channels. This can never be done as long as we deny the existence of anger. The dangerous person is not the angry person. The dangerous person is one who is angry and does not know it. To look honestly in the mirror may bring the discovery of a surprising amount of anger. If you discover anger, recognize it, claim it, and deal with it.

Another possibility is that honest self-analysis may also allow frustration to surface. While frustration may be similar to anger, it becomes significant as it describes our response to goals and dreams that just did not work out. An honest appraisal of ourselves may reveal that we are not where we thought we would be.

We may not have failed outright, but we surely did not make it as we thought. One reason persons of middle age are prone to the self-insulating attempts of hyperactivity may be the realization that it just hasn't worked out according to plan. The truth is that very few persons are where they hoped to be. Frustration is the natural response to dreams that fall short. The chances are quite likely that frustration may be a part of your own agenda. Denying it, once again, becomes a vicious cycle. Frustration calls for a time of reevaluation and reassessment. A wise person will make new goals and continue to dream new dreams. Which brings to mind another likely discovery.

We also will find that change is inevitable. To look honestly at ourselves reminds us that we are not the same, our friends are not the same, and our circumstances are not the same. Generally speaking, we do not like change; but it comes in many forms. To quote my friend Bob once again: "Self-talk became a part of my healing. I told myself time and again to acknowledge and accept my vulnerability to life's uncertainties, risks, and tragedies—even joys. And no one is exempt."

If change is inevitable, then so is the vulnerability that

follows. Some of the change within and without cannot be altered. Yet, we do have the opportunity to influence the flow of some things. One fact is certain: We cannot redirect the flow of anything as long as we deny the reality of change. Hair coloring can cover the changing years only so long. Face up to change and discover the simple beauty of gray hair. One cannot discover the touch of God's hand upon senior adult days unless one admits that senior adulthood is a reality. Change is inevitable. Accept it, and get on with the next phase of the journey.

Life is one long process of saying hello and good-bye. These are among the first words we learn as children, and they continue to be part of our language. Learning how and when to say hello and good-bye facilitates learning how to rest.

Many discoveries can be made that are exciting and affirming. Honesty is not just a negative experience. But, none of these discoveries can be made as long as one frantically avoids oneself.

There are some forces in life from which we should run. To place ourselves, however, in such company is foolish indeed. The reason is obvious. To flee a robber on a dark street may be wise when there is room to run. But, where is our retreat when we flee from ourselves? There is nowhere to go.

Restlessness is the inevitable result of avoiding oneself. Discovering peace with God and peace with oneself are natural requirements for genuine rest. Otherwise, rest never comes. Some may spend a lifetime running and so much is missed along the way. Others may be forced by illness or injury to look inside themselves. Some, however, may be wise enough to realize that avoiding oneself is just plain stupid.

Drop thy still dews of quietness,
   Till all our strivings cease;
Take from our souls the strain and stress,
   And let our ordered lives confess
The beauty of thy peace.
            —John Greenleaf Whittier

7

Dealing with Our Compulsiveness

Our ability to rest is quite frequently influenced by the makeup of our own personalities. Some people by the nature of their personalities are more likely to relax than others. Each of us has traits that place us in at least one of several general personality groups even though there is risk involved in reducing complex human nature into a single type. One's personality refers to those characteristic and distinctive traits of an individual.

While there are many similarities from one personality to another, there are some distinct and interesting differences. Henry Murray said "People is mostly alike, but what difference they is can be powerful important." One difference is that some personality types have more difficulty resting than others.

One type, in particular, which finds rest a frustrating challenge is the compulsive personality. Such a person has an irresistible impulse to act, and the goal is nothing less than total perfection. Some of us experience this type in varying degrees. The compulsive person is not necessarily neurotic or psychotic but does have the endless task of keeping everything in its rightful place. Organization and complete order are demanded before this person can relax. She may make a super administrator and good manager but the ability to relax and rest is not her long suit. After all, when does one ever position oneself to rest when perfection is necessary before one has the right to relax?

The compulsive person is not always the neurotic who may be out of touch with reality. Instead, this individual is the perfectionist who simply wants things done right. The desire for order and quality is admirable for any person; but if absolute perfection is required before one can temporarily retire, the opportunities for rest become practically nonexistent. How often is everything just as it should be? Very seldom!

Therefore, we are forced to learn how to rest in spite of the fact that everything is not just like we want it. For some, the process of resting when everything is not according to the predetermined plan is an awesome challenge. We must resign ourselves to the fact that we are limited creatures and live in an imperfect world. We can do only so much to make everything work according to plan. If rest is the reward for perfection, we will quickly become angry, tired, and frustrated.

Regardless of our particular endeavor, perfection is a continuum upon which we travel and hope to progress. Rest is precisely the discipline that allows us to continue the process and not a reward that comes to us at the end of the journey. Rest is not the end of our pursuits. It is the means by which we mentally, emotionally, physically, and spiritually equip ourselves to accomplish the tasks placed before us. If rest is granted as a consequence of perfection, it should be to prepare for the next venture.

Accepting the limited nature of our own mortality is not an easy task for some people. For various reasons we have images of our capabilities that are self-defeating and place great and needless demands upon us. Life contains too many variables for us to be totally in control. The excessive need to compulsively control one's surroundings is a very difficult way to do the business of life.

The opposite is not apathy and insensitivity. By nature and accomplishment we are granted the opportunities to bring about change. The beauty of the human experience is found at the very point of change and progress. To ignore the opportunities for the bettering of one's surroundings is sin indeed. The problem comes when we cross over the line from some control to total control. There is a difference. One is admirable. The other is unhealthy.

The purpose of these few pages is not to give a technical treatment of the obsessive-compulsive disorder. Such a disorder is a very serious matter and is far too complex to deal with in a few paragraphs. The issue being raised at this point is that many of us have some rather compulsive behavioral habits which, if ignored, can seriously impede effective resting.

Obsessive thoughts and compulsive urges or actions are a part of everyday life. We return to check a locked door before we go to bed. We check several times to make certain the stove is shut off. We practice the speech we are to make to the civic club next week.

Only when these thoughts or rituals become so frequent or extensive that they interfere with normal functioning is the diagnosis of obsessive-compulsive disorder made. While most of us fall short of the diagnosis, we possess enough of a perfectionist nature to create for ourselves a great deal of anxiety and discomfort.

Compulsions are defined as: "Repetitive and seemingly purposeful behaviors that are performed according to certain rules or in a stereotyped fashion. The behavior is not an end in itself, but is designed to produce or prevent some future event or situation. However, either the activity is not connected in a realistic way with what it is designed to produce or prevent or it may be clearly excessive."[1]

Textbook cases of obsessive-compulsive disorders are relatively rare. In fact, traditional estimates of such cases in the general population are as low as 0.05 percent. Therefore, while we may possess some perfectionistic habits, we are far from being psychotic. For the compulsive man or woman, however, rest may be an awesome challenge. The achievement of perfection is a rare experience for most of us. Somehow we must develop the ability to find peace and relaxation at a point less than perfect.

One significant area of anxiety for us may not be in regard to things but in regard to people and more specifically in the way we relate to people. Frequently our compulsive behavior finds expression in the way we try to control others. Sometimes our desire to control is a result of good and honorable intentions. On other occasions selfish desires become the reason. Sigmund Freud once described a part of the maturing process as learning to accept the differentness of others.

A strong case could be made to prove that one of the most irresistible temptations to misuse power is the temptation to take control of other people's lives. Wives do it. Husbands do it. Parents do it. Siblings do it. Politicians do it. Friends do it, and on and on. Most of us have enough difficulty controlling our own lives. How can we possibly control the circumstances surrounding someone else?

The person who is compelled to control other people will find rest a rare experience.

The temptation to control is real and ongoing for all of us, especially in our relationships with people who are closest to us. Husbands and wives, for example, have many ways of trying to control and manipulate one another. The manipulated one finds difficulty in experiencing personal growth through the exercise of his or her own special gifts.

The compulsive controller presumes that the person being controlled will never be big enough and smart enough to make adequate decisions and choices. The temptation is to take over the control of those persons with whom one has regular contact because they are seen as indecisive and immature. To relate to people in such a way requires a tremendous amount of work, possibly endless work.

One's professional role may require the supervision and management of many individuals. But even then management does not necessarily equal control. As a parent one is charged with the ultimate care of children. Still, healthy parenting does not necessarily equal control.

When manipulation is at the base of our relationship, we not only have to work endless overtime hours but also lose the joy of relationships. A loving relationship is based on the willingness of each of the parties to call forth the unique, God-given gifts of the other. The desire to manipulate and control is a contradiction of this essential ingredient.

God created us in His own image and yet granted us the freedom to express our human nature in very unique ways. Why can we not grant our associates the same privilege? To exercise power over people around us not only denies them the opportunity to express their own uniqueness but also denies us the opportunity to experience the joy of differentness. The need to control denies another's personal integrity.

Consider all the time and energy required to make everything work out according to our plans. Procrustes, of Greek mythology, embodies the extreme case of one who is compulsively determined to make everyone fit according to his plan. When guests visited Procrustes overnight, he invited them to sleep in the Procrustean bed. If they were too short for the bed, Procrustes stretched them to fit. If they were too long for the bed, Procrustes cut off their legs to make them fit. From this character comes the word *Procrusteanism.* The Procrustean person is one who insists on everyone conforming precisely to his or her concept of what one should be. A tremendous amount of work is involved in making everyone fit a certain mold.

The most loving thing we can do for the persons who are close to us is to affirm their unique gifts. In fact, Dr. Anthony Campolo, in a lecture delivered to the Furman Pastor's School, indicated that we cannot love someone and exercise power over them at the same time. In his lecture and his book, *The Power Delusion,* he offered a very unique understanding of the relationship of power and love. The exercising of power adversely affects one's ability to love.

Occasionally we try to control others because they threaten our own inadequacy. When we are easily threatened by others, we can find little joy and no peace. Therefore, we work overtime trying to maintain control over those about us in order to lessen our feelings of insecurity.

The essence of Christian love is giving oneself to others so that they can be fulfilled and affirmed. Recreating them in our image precludes that opportunity. Trying to play God with the lives of others requires a high price of ener-

gy from us. Such a need diminishes our joy, our spontanei-
ty, and our rest. We are seldom the master of our own fate,
much less that of anyone else.

The desire to be in full control was man's original problem. How long does it take us to learn that such a need is
very expensive in many ways? The compulsive need to
regenerate people in our own image and totally control
our circumstances is a great inhibitor of peace and rest.

Note

1. Michael A. Jenike, Lee Baer, and William Menichiello, eds.,
Obsessive Compulsive Disorders (Littleton, Mass.: P. S. G. Pub-
lishing Company, Inc.,), p. 2.

8

Noise Within and Without

Any attempt to deal with our problems of unrest must
include consideration of the noise which surrounds most
of us. Our world is basically noisy, at least for the majority
of us. Think of the last time you heard nothing. That's
right, absolutely nothing. Many of us are extremely uncomfortable with the sound of nothingness. We don't
know what to do with it. One reason for our uneasiness is
that such a sound occurs so seldom. There are few opportunities for silence. Living in our world today requires
much from us. We must continually make adjustments.
We need fresh perspectives. We need clear judgment. We
need a renewing of our energies. And many of these
needs cannot be met in the noise of a battle. An interna-
tional retreat into the gentle arms of silence soothes like
medicine to the wounded.

I can remember when we, many years ago, began to
hear references to noise pollution. From a relatively small
town in south Georgia, I associated noise pollution with
big cities, airports, and interstate highways. My personal

impression at the time was that a big fuss was being made over nothing. Big city sounds were a world away. If I wanted silence, all I had to do was to visit my grandmother in the country. A young boy has no passion for silence. Quiet is what your dad wants when he feels you have said enough. Silence means there is nothing going on, so I thought then. In one's youth, noise means action. Now noise surrounds most of us whether we are city or country folk. At times we would pay a high price for some of that quiet which was such a bore to us as children.

Try to seek a place of quiet and discover how difficult such a task is. For those of us who live in the city, silence seems to be an impossible goal. Regardless of where we live, however, there are opportunities for solitude if we honestly search for such a place. We do not have to go deep into a nationally protected forest to discover a place of quiet. Solitude may be as close as our own backyard. Solitude enhances genuine rest. We do not need to remain in the realm of the quiet. Retreat has value only when the setting provides a needed contrast. Occasional periods of silence are vital for the renewing of our physical, mental, and spiritual strength. Surely one of the reasons for the confused state of many people today is the difficulty and scarcity of solitude. Possibly we have just forgotten how important it is.

I occasionally seek the solitude of the ocean and a quiet beach. Even the mesmerizing sound of the ocean can make its share of noise. But, for a beach lover like me that noise enters my body like a tranquilizer. The fact that our body subconsciously responds to this soothing sound should remind us that we are receptors of the sounds all around us. We are constantly responding to what we hear, whether we are aware of it or not.

The desire for silence causes us to be more conscious of

the sounds all about us. Noise will then create a certain amount of rage within us when our silence is invaded. My family and I took a vacation at the beach recently. The hypnotic rhythm of the ocean seemed to be the perfect prescription for getting some writing done. I planted myself on a rather quiet section of beach. The only sounds I could hear were from the surf and the wind. Anyone can become a philosopher in such a setting, and many of us have tried it at some time. My philosophizing soon gave way to gentle, beautiful sleep. I had hardly gone to sleep when I was startled awake by the sounds of a entire rock band playing somewhere around my chair. As I came to my senses, I realized that the noise was coming from a "dual-speakered, dual-decked, dual-equalized radio with a handle" carried by a young girl walking the beach. My first impulse was to throw her noise box in the ocean, but I feared that her daddy was a frustrated karate instructor and that he was back at his motel waiting for the chance to practice his art.

Noise had invaded my rest. I felt very frustrated. And that experience is relived nearly every day for most of us. There are very few opportunities for most of us to experience silence. And when we have a chance we usually manufacture some kind of noise. Silence may force us to deal with ourselves which is the very person some of us will avoid at all costs.

Allow me another personal experience to make a point, even if trite. Something happened recently that borders on a real crisis. The radio in my car died. Wheels and brakes one can do without, but a radio is a neccessity. I try to use my radio wisely. I listen to a variety of music, including the classics, religious music, and an occasional Bill Cosby tape. My work requires that I spend a lot of time in my car, and a good radio becomes a close companion. The manufacturer agreed to repair the radio if I returned it. But, that would mean days without it. Laugh if you like, but the quietness of my car required some adjustment.

Surprisingly, I found myself enjoying the silence. I began to notice certain sounds outside the car of which I otherwise would be unaware. The quiet solitude of an automobile can become a quiet beach for all kinds of philosophizing. Fortunately, I usually can manage to stay awake.

One morning recently I was driving to the office. The hour was early, and I was using the time for personal meditation, which I believe makes a lot more sense than shouting at other drivers during rush hour traffic. As I stopped at a traffic light, a truck pulled up beside me. He had a radio playing so loud that it could have been heard in South America. The windows were rolled up, and the entire truck body vibrated with the pounding beat of the music. I am no prude and have played music loud in my day, but come on!

My first impulse was to break his windows to see if he would even notice but he appeared to be stronger and in better shape than I was so I restrained myself. I could not help but wonder what effect all of that noise was having on his emotional state. Our bodies cannot be unaffected by the sounds all around us. Although one person's music may be another one's noise, we are constantly responding to the sounds all around us.

Dr. Wayne Hodges, a neurologist in Savannah, Georgia, has offered an interesting opinion in regard to our body's response to sight and sound. Dr. Hodges does not believe in the subconscious, at least in the traditional style of Freud or Jung. The subconscious is not some strange mysterious part of the brain but rather a process of sensory data being passed from outside the body to the hypothalamus without the direct involvement of the forebrain. Dr. Hodges explains how through classical training (the development of habits) our bodies develop the ability to respond to light and sound without the direct involvement of our conscious process, the forebrain. The subconscious becomes the process of sensory data passing straight to the interbrain which then creates the appropriate reaction from our body, frequently without a conscious mental awareness.

My intent is not to promote a particular theory of the subconscious but to make a point. The point is quite simple. Our bodies are constantly responding to the sounds all around us whether we are aware of them or not. Noise pollution is a problem. Our bodies cry out for rest and also for an environment that makes rest possible. How can we possibly rest when our sensory system is continually bombarded with sight and sound that calls for a response. We may want rest, but we do not give our mental and physical systems much of an opportunity. A break from the constant sensory overload is necessary.

Dr. Wayne Oates has written a marvelous book entitled _Nurturing Silence in a Noisy Heart,_ which should be listed as a classic for anyone honestly searching for a place of restful silence. Dr. Oates has, in his insightful way, called attention to the fact that silence must be cultivated. "If you and I ever have silence in our noisy hearts, we are going to have to grow it. . . . You can nurture silence in you noisy hearts if you value it, cherish it, and are eager to nourish it . . ."[1]

The revitalizing of our energies depends upon occasional retreats into silence. We should never be afraid of it. Solitude is a friend. An anonymous poet has written:

There is a voice, "a still, small voice" of love,
     Heard from above;
But not amidst the din of earthly sounds,
     Which here confounds:
By those withdrawn apart it best is heard,
And peace, sweet peace, breathes in each gentle word.

My favorite psalm is Psalm 46. One reason for the power of these words for me is that they expose the truth of my life-style. The psalmist very clearly instructed us to "be still, and know." For the psalmist, "knowing God" was much more than an intellectual exercise. Knowing God strikes at one's deepest needs for assurance and security. But, to "know" one must first be still.

Many explanations have been offered as to the background of this psalm. Some have suggested that the words were a response to the assault of the Assyrian army. The battering rams of Sennacherib's forces had overpowered everything in their path. One cannot read these stirring words without sensing the writer's fatigue. That fatigue occurred amid great noise.

Notice the carefully chosen words. "The earth be removed. . . . mountains shake." Do you hear the noise of the psalmist's world? Do you sense his fatigue? It was no accident that he began and ended his words with a reference to God as strength and refuge.

The solution to his troubled and noisy world was quite simple. One is to look to the God of refuge and strength. How is God to be found? "Be still, and know. . . ."

The noise of our world is not in the battering rams of the Assyrian army. But the noise is there just the same. Our noise is experienced through a hurried life-style, countless demands, and the frustration of never accomplishing what seems to be enough.

Consider the example of Jesus. Surely we can learn

much from the way He conducted His life. Jesus was a man, but not an ordinary man. As the Son of God, Jesus possessed powers which are foreign to an average person. Yet, in His humanity we can observe a man who periodically needed to get away and rest in silence. Scripture records many occasions when Jesus had to get away from all the demands placed upon Him and allow silence to embrace Him.

If Jesus, the Son of God, had needs that could only be met in solitude, how can we possibly assume to function without the same? As great as His love was for people, He would periodically slip away from the noise of the maddening crowd. He understood clearly the instruction of the psalmist to "be still, and know." One can offer many suggestions for the unusual strength of Jesus. High on that list must be the periodic times of retreat when Jesus slipped away from the noise of His world. The need for deep physical and spiritual breaths in moments of silence cannot be ignored.

Generally speaking, the noise of our world is necessary. One would be foolish to think that he or she could live in continuous silence. Factories produce goods necessary for our existence. Highways guide us from place to place. Construction sites are a sign of growth. And who would want to deny the noise of a Friday evening football game in the fall? However, fatigue has the power to turn opportunities into curses. Unless one periodically turns aside from the noise, normal demands can become overwhelming.

One other observation must be shared at this point. Just as we must deal with the noise of the world without as we seek rest, we also must deal with the noise within us. Many sources of noise within directly relate to our unrest. Allow me to briefly mention three, although the list could be very long. First, there is the noise of guilt. Guilt is a universal problem. Guilt gnaws at our stomachs and turns in our head at night. How difficult it is to sit still and relax when we have royally fouled up! Whether anyone else knows it or not does not matter. We know it, and that is enough.

In fact, some of our most difficult moments of guilt are when we alone know of our shortcoming. The only thing worse than being found out is the fear of being found out. The Bible wisely describes, "The wicked flee when no one pursues" (Prov. 28:1).

Guilt is a noise within us which can seriously inhibit our rest. Is there a person anywhere who has not tossed during the night amid the pangs of guilt? A deed, a word, or a misunderstanding turns over and over in our mind, and there is no rest for the weary. The noise of unresolved guilt cannot be ignored.

Only one solution can be found. Guilt must be honestly and directly resolved. Guilt is a triangle, and one must touch all three corners which include others, God, and self. To change the noise of guilt into restful silence, one must direct oneself to all three corners in the appropriate order. The Bible speaks very clearly to the fact that if we have "aught" with our brother we should go to him before we approach God's altar. *Aught* is not a commonly used word in our modern language, but the meaning is clear. If you have wronged someone, go straight to that person. Deliver your mail to the right house. Seek forgiveness from your neighbor first. Then, you are ready to approach God. As important as God's forgiveness is, it will never be a way of avoiding our neighbor. God's forgiveness is not an escape from reality.

The next corner of the triangle is God. God's forgiveness is not just a nice idea. Forgiveness is an event, some-

thing that really happens. Once forgiveness has been received, let it be done. There is no value in continuing to
carry the guilt. When you carry the trash out of your
house, you do not bring it back into the house when you
return. Just as foolish is the process of asking for God's
forgiveness and then continuing to carry around a load of
guilt.

The third corner of the triangle must not be ignored if
you are to discover peace. You must be willing to forgive
yourself. In all reality the most difficult dimension of forgiveness may be the task of dealing with yourself. The
forgiveness of your neighbor and of God can bring you
little joy if you refuse to grant the same forgiving spirit to
yourself.

Christ has already climbed a cruel cross once. There is
no need for that experience to be relived in our own lives.
To refuse to grant forgiveness to ourselves weakens the
forgiving power of the cross of Jesus. Yet some of us will
attempt to personally relive the cross over and over again.
If you cannot forgive yourself, and release in a very private and personal way the guilt you carry, you might
consider sharing this problem with someone trained for
and sensitive to such a problem. Begin with your minister,
but be honest. Games are self-defeating.

Second, consider the noise that exists within us due to
anger. Anger is a powerful emotion and should never be
ignored. Anger which is ignored becomes master of the
soul. And so many people seem angry these days!

Recently I was driving on a busy, six-lane street in
Augusta. A young woman wanted to enter the traffic from
a parking lot. The traffic was moving slow, so I let her in
front of me. There was a temporary opening in the lane
to my right and she went over into that lane also. When
she did, the man in front of whom she pulled exploded

into a tirade, swinging his fists, and hurling curses that were quite creative. His shouts could be heard above all the rush-hour noise.

The man's actions were not entertaining at all. His case was very sad to me. He must be a very angry person to have been outraged by such an insignificant event. If letting another driver in front of him in traffic erupts that much emotion, his inner world must be a noisy one.

So much frustration exists among people today, and anger is an inevitable element of frustration. The poor handling of anger accounts for much of our social pathology, from physical abuse and other forms of violence all the way to deep-seated depression. Anger is a dynamic which is far too complicated to deal with in a few sentences. The need exists for a great deal of study of the "angry person" in our culture. For present purposes, let me make just a few observations as to the lessening of the inner noise of anger.

First, if you are angry, do not deny it. If there is one person who concerns me more than the angry person, it is the person who is angry and does not know it. Anger which is denied sits in the driver's seat.

Second, confess your anger to a trusted friend or colleague. Talking honestly with someone about your feelings can take some of the sting out of the emotion. An understanding but calming friend can frequently keep us out of some very embarrassing situations.

Third, become sensitive to what anger may cause you to do. When anger is sitting under our emotional steering wheel, we can say and do some very cruel things. Later on we may ask why in the world we did such a thing. A moment of honesty reveals the truth. "We were mad." Be sensitive to words and deeds whose origin may have been in the realm of blind anger rather than mature reason.

Fourth, try to look beyond the immediate event. Our feelings may have been hurt, but, ultimately, what bearing will it have on the outcome? Some things are worthy of our anger, but not everything. Try to back away from the heat for a moment to get a better perspective. Yes, right now what was said or done may hurt. But, will it, ultimately, make much difference? One sign of maturity is the realization that some things are worthy of our anger and some are not.

Anger is a noise that has interrupted the rest of many weary souls. If anger is a serious problem for you, do not ignore its impact upon your life. Deal with it, honestly and directly.

For the sake of time and space, I will mention only one other noise within us. Consider the interruptive powers of discontentment. Effective rest demands a "settling in" on the present moment. We can never claim the present moment when our discontentment forces us to live in another time and place. Most of us spend too many of our days and nights wishing we were someone else, living somewhere else, and in some other time frame. How can we ever relax when our immediate circumstances provide no joy?

The opposite of discontentment is not complacency. The opposite is a sense of acceptance and openness. The key to silencing the noise of discontentment is the healthy acceptance of self and circumstance. Acceptance does not rule out the excitement of bettering one's self and circumstance. In order to improve, however, you must begin where you are. You cannot start "over there." You begin with things as they are.

Discontentment is a thief. It robs us of gentle smiles, sweet smells, and momentary sights. Paul said, "I have learned in whatever state I am, to be content. . . . I have learned both to be full and to be hungry, both to abound and to suffer need" (Phil. 4: 11-12). Because of his personal discipline the chances are good that Paul rested quite well at night. There seemed to be very little noise of discontentment.

Our world is a noisy one. The noise is within and without. How desparately many of us need recreative moments of solitude and silence. Silence is not just the absence of noise. Silence is something we experience. Silence is not passive. It is active involvement in the nurturing of a need of the human soul. Noise within and without inhibits the renewing of our energies. Quiet moments sooth our soul and enlarge our vision. Silence is not an enemy. It is a friend. Do not be afraid of it. "Be still, and know. . . ."

Note

1. Wayne E. Oates, *Nurturing Silence in a Noisy Heart* (Garden City, N.Y.: Doubleday and Company, Inc., 1979), p. 3.

9

Productivity and the Work Ethic

By definition the work-rest cycle implies continuity from one part to the other. Therefore, a poor concept of work will inherently influence one's concept of rest. Easy movement from one to the other is not always the case with some of us. There may be work and rest in one's schedule, but neither is very pleasant nor meaningful.

At the risk of oversimplification consider the example of an automobile tire. Due to poor maintenance several flat spots are created in the tire. The tire still rolls, continues to function, and can still be considered a tire. But, the ride is rough, noisy, and generally unpleasant. The same can happen to our work and our rest.

Rest has little meaning when it bears no relationship to work. They directly influence each other, and one of the "flat spots" which frequently occurs in the cycle is the result of a poor or inadequate concept of work. Any discussion of work should take into consideration the impact of the old Protestant ethic. A brief look at the Protestant (work) ethic is worthy of our time at this point.

In early America one had no choice but to work for economic survival. The economic necessity for work soon developed moral implications as well. This moral obligation became the basis for what is referred to as the Protestant ethic.

The American attitudes toward work were drastically affected by the powerful and competing movements of the Reformation and the Enlightenment. Both were primarily reactions against the traditional church but carried forceful messages concerning the individual and his work.

The Reformation began with Martin Luther in the fifteenth century. One strong tenet of Luther was that there was no virtue in poverty. He envisioned mankind as being in the world to serve God and others. In the process of serving there was nothing inherently evil about wealth, only the wrong use of it. A moral person will, therefore, not lose himself to wealth and will use it for the good of all people.

He held to the unusual concept of a worldly calling. This calling was to be seen in contrast with the high calling of the monastic life of the Roman Catholic Church. This secular calling of Luther was to be seen also in contrast with the old concept of work as a curse which had been prevalent for centuries. Labor, interestingly, became more than atonement for original sin. Work had significance and was seen as a bridge between earth and heaven.

John Calvin carried the concept one step further by preaching maximum effort. "When a person produces more than he needs," said Calvin, "this surplus should not be wasted on personal appetites. It should serve the glory of God by being reinvested to improve one's work and provide even greater surpluses for the glory of God."[1]

A major shift also occurred in the general attitude toward profit making. For centuries the Christian church condemned profit making, associating wealth primarily with the role of the oppressor. Suddenly wealth was understood as a sign of God's blessing. One was not only granted the moral opportunity to work but also given the go ahead to make a profit. Remember, however, that the profit was to serve the glory of God.

Underlying the Protestant ethic was the belief that people do not work for themselves alone. The calling comes from God, and people prove their worth to themselves and to God by their dedicated labors.

Also underlying this concept was the belief that work is good. One of the by-products of the ethic was an emphasis on thrift and specific discouragement of spending large amounts of money on personal pleasures. Unnecessary luxuries were seen as a distraction from duties to God.

According to the ethic, one is good and virtuous if one is hard-working and thrifty. One who is lazy and wasteful would not be affirmed. The concept placed great emphasis on personal responsibility. The end result of dedication and hard work was success.

Max Weber, a German sociologist, in 1904 wrote a famous essay, "The Protestant Ethic and the Spirit of Capitalism." He proposed that the principles of the Protestant ethic contributed to the advancement of the economic system called capitalism. Capitalism maintains that the competition of individuals for wealth through work helps to build a strong economy.

Two hundred years after the time of Luther and Calvin, John Wesley began to point to the negative outcome of the Protestant ethic. There could be little question that such an expression of faith would produce industry and frugality which would result in wealth. Unfortunately, as riches increase so would pride, anger, and desire. The system, Wesley predicted, would bring about its own downfall. To avoid such an outcome he strongly encouraged people to share their wealth so they would grow in grace.

The influence of the Protestant ethic and the wisdom of Wesley's forsight is obvious. Wealth did increase in America, and riches became the symbol of respectability. Riches became an end in itself rather than a way of glorifying God. Wealth was no longer a means of growing in God's grace but a goal in and of itself. Material success became the ultimate aspiration.

The concept of spiritaual calling in one's work became history. An industrialized society had little sympathy for such a belief. The objective of work was economic gain. People caught in an industrialized environment became very frustrated and found very little meaning in their work. They experienced even less prestige. The result of all of these changing attitudes toward work is still with us today, and we cannot ignore its influence.

Many workers realized that, regardless of how hard they worked, they would never attain economic success. To compensate for their strong feelings of monotony and frustration, greater demands were made for more financial compensation. Their work activity had little meaning apart from the paycheck, which was never enough to suffice. Meaning was not to be found in their response to God's calling them to their jobs, but only in the compensation that was produced.

The twentieth century brought about a change from the Protestant ethic to a consumption ethic. The Protestant ethic encouraged people to work hard and save their money. The heart of consumerism is to work as little as possible and spend the money as quickly as possible since it will not be worth as much tomorrow. The Protestant ethic taught people to save their money for the future, but the consumer ethic encourages attention to the present, frequently at the expense of the future. Demand your reward now!

Just as was predicted by Wesley and others, the Protestant ethic came to support a system that eventually self-destructed. In today's culture one of the real dangers of our present economic system is that it has no moral and spiritual foundation. While we can easily recognize the influence of the Protestant ethic on our modern economic culture, it is no longer the predominant influence on attitudes about work in our society. Unfortunately, we live in the world of consumerism. Make as much as you can, as quickly as you can, and spend it as fast as you can.

What does all of this have to do with rest? Our concept of work has a very direct effect on the quality of our rest. The cycle functions better with healthy attitudes toward work and rest. The quality of our rest improves as we find meaning and fulfillment in our work. Meaningless work creates the conditions for a restlessness which permeates all that we do.

A very practical issue exists as well. When we find meaning in our work, we will make a more conscious effort in our rest habits. We want to do well when we have a reason for our work. We are willing to give time to rest so that we might operate at our best.

There are some lingering spin-offs from the old Protestant ethic. Needless to say, profit making is still acceptable today, although the motivation has little to do with glorifying God. Profits are not inherently evil since no business can operate long without them. We have also accepted the belief that it is commendable to make more than we need. Yet, when we have no sense of calling to our job, our paycheck becomes our single reward. Such a utilitarian system is quite risky.

For example, what are the people to do who know that their wages will always be minimal? Let's be honest, not everyone can earn the big salary. If being at peace with ourselves in relation to our work depends solely on the paycheck, many people are destined for restlessness.

With the enslaving entrance of television into our lives, the whole world knows how wealthy people live and the assumption is that everyone is supposed to live like that. The typical television drama and sitcom pictures the American family as having almost everything one could want. As cute and funny as Bill Cosby's television program might be, not every family has a lawyer mother and a doctor father and plenty of time for leisurely conversation. The majority of American people will never know that kind of life-style. Someone must continue to oil the wheels of industry, and frequently the financial results are far less than the image offered by television. A meaningful concept of work must make room for more than just a paycheck.

Allow me to offer a personal observation to illustrate my point. I grew up in a mill town where the textitle industry dominated everyone's life. After college and seminary I served as an industrial chaplain for a textile firm. Therefore, for many years I have had the opportunity to observe some of God's best people, mill folk.

I have watched them tend a machine for so many hours that they have little time for fun and frolic. In many cases the work is hard and quite monotonous. Why do they stay with it? How can they continue to go through the same motions shift after shift? For some the reward may be a larger paycheck than they could make at another semi-skilled job. In most cases the financial reward is just not that great and, as a result, the turnover is quite significant. Some, however, have managed to discover meaning in what they do.

Consider Mr. Brooks who tends a spinning frame. He works six and sometimes seven days a week and will double if given the chance. His job would bore most people. Mr. Brooks cannot read or write, but his hourly wage is paying for his daughter to go to nursing school. Mr. Brooks is proud of his job because it is his daughter's ticket to the future.

Consider Mrs. Jones who works in the light house and inspects hundreds of cones of yarn every day. Most people would have tired long ago of looking at the endless line of cones under the light. But, what you need to know is that Mrs. Jones is an alcoholic who lost practically everything. The job she now has was offered to her by a sensitive shift manager who believed in her. For Mrs. Jones her paycheck is secondary to her restored personal dignity.

In the two cases and many others like them, people have carved out of their routine jobs a reason for it all. I also have an idea that they sleep well at night because there is meaning to their life, something beyond their compensation. They rest well because they want to do their best and a reason undergirds their work.

When a paycheck becomes our sole reward for our labor, we have set sail on an endless and usually fruitless pursuit for peace and happiness. The main problem lies in the obvious characteristic of our human nature: Enough is never enough! How many people do you know who have enough? A business colleague of my father once said that there were only two pieces of property he wanted, his and the one next to it. Buying up the world does not leave much time for rest. The rich may get richer, but they are seldom satisfied. Rest is hard to find.

Our society can be described as operating within a consumeristic system. The biggest fallacy with consumerism is that we can never buy enough to provide meaning for our lives. There is always a bigger house, a more expensive car, and an endless array of adult toys. The sad truth is that the more we have the more restless we become. There is always someone who can out buy us. If we relax, we might lose our symbols of success and drop down a few notches on the status-conscious ladder of success.

One dynamic of the Protestant ethic is still at work in many of our attitudes about work. One of the attitudes stressed in the ethic emphasizes that people prove their worth to themselves and to God by dedicated achievement. In other words, one's value is determined by what can be produced. Measuring our worth by what we can produce is risky business. Several problems may result. How does one find worth if some disability prevents physical labor? When one retires, does one step out of a job and self-worth?

If our value is secured by our work, the temptation is great to produce more and more to increase our worth. A logical spin-off is that we push ourselves beyond our limits in our efforts to feel good about ourselves. Paul wrote that if a man does not work he should not eat. Work is honorable, desirable, and a part of God's plan. But, work does not make of us persons of worth. The end result of such a strategy is a painful, vicious cycle.

I have to believe that my worth comes from the One in whose image I have been created. Holy Scripture describes Jesus as having a "name which is above every name" (Phil. 2:9). Our name may not be above every name but it is, indeed, a name! My value comes not from my time card or production report but from the One who created me.

Even though the old Protestant ethic may have traveled a course of self-destruction, one of its primary attitudes would serve us well if recaptured. There is room today for a sense of spiritual calling or secular calling to our work. Dr. Vicktor Frankl discovered in the Nazi concentration camps that one can endure almost anything if meaning can be found. The most routine job can be endured and even enjoyed if meaning undergirds the process.

Most workers today experience little or no sense of calling to their work. Their attachment is found only in the convenience of their job, the pay scale, or the lack of any other option. The inevitable result is a painful sense of restlessness. No amount of physical rest can send one with a smile to one's job on Monday morning if the motivation is only to avoid poverty.

In Japan the work ethic has had a particularly interesting effect on rest. In Japan the work ethic is so strong that managers have a problem with workers not taking vacations. When forced to take vacations, many workers feel so much guilt that they cannot achieve rest. Some Japanese companies have recognized this as a significant social problem and are establishing programs to help Japanese professionals learn how to use vacation time without feeling guilty.

In America, however, the Protestant ethic is gone forever. While it may have indirectly set into motion forces that are sources of problems for our society, we would do well to recapture the sense of meaning that the ethic can provide for our work.

Note

1. Perry Pascarella, *The New Achievers* (New York: The Free Press,), p. 30.

10

The Effects of
Stress upon Rest

Allow your imagination to work for a moment and determine if the following experience is familiar to you. Imagine that you have been looking forward to some vacation time for a long while. Friday afternoon has finally arrived, and you are on your way home. As usual, the traffic is extremely heavy; you are forced to make those periodic stops. Moving slowly in the traffic, you think about all the leisure hours of the week that is to come. No traffic, no demands, and no schedule to keep. The problems of the job will be far away, and the only decisions you plan to make in the next seven days will be deciding what to eat, when to sleep, and where to nap.

You like to think that deep inside you are made for the leisure life and just have not been given the opportunity to express that side of your personality. You finally arrive home and think to yourself with a great sigh, *Friday night has arrived, the beginning of the week for which I have lived since last year's vacation week.* The unwinding process will take only a few minutes, and then rest and relaxation will be the name of the game. However, at the moment you have a little trouble sitting still.

The newspaper does not seem very interesting, and the chair just does not sit well at the moment. While watching television, you are reminded of some things that really needed to be done at work but 5:00 PM came so quickly. As you go to bed, you remember that the alarm clock can be ignored tonight. Of all nights you cannot go to sleep. You toss and turn and try to remember that tomorrow morning brings no demands, no struggles, no confrontations. Sleep finally comes, and you wake up earlier than you normally would. You try to go back to sleep, which on any other morning you would give your eyeteeth for the chance, but this morning your eyes are locked open. Out of frustration you get up. Today will be a day of total relaxation! Since you didn't sleep well, an extra nap will be in order for the morning.

The newspaper and a cup of coffee will start the day and vacation time in proper fashion. You start to sit down and notice the trash has filled the canister in the kitchen, and no one wants to look at last night's remains. If you take it outside, you can then settle down to some serious newspaper reading.

As you start to make the coffee, you notice that the percolator really could use some scrubbing. After all, it has not been cleaned since your mother-in-law, out of fear, scrubbed it last Christmas. The coffee would taste better, anyway. How benevolent you are to do this not only for yourself but also for everyone else in the family! As you lift that first symbolic cup of coffee on this, your long-awaited vacation week, you suddenly remember one matter that really should have been completed yesterday before you left work but in the rush you totally forgot. If you can clear this one matter, you will not think of the job for a whole week. In fact, you make a promise to yourself that during the next seven days you will not even let thoughts of the job cross your mind. The telephone call is made and all is well, finally. The coffee is cold. You pour another and sit down, but you cannot remember what you did with the newspaper. It is not by the telephone. Surely you did not drop it in the trash earlier. You go outside and check the can. Just as you guessed, there it is and beautifully decorated with last night's food scraps. Back to the coffee that is cold again. Enough is enough. Forget the leisurely morning and plans for an extra nap. The lawn needs to be mowed. After all, even vacation weeks need to be productive.

If you can relate to this experience, you are not alone and you are also familiar with stress. Most of us are not aware of the long-term effects of stress upon our lives, particularly the silent, lingering effects. Stress is not just the great moments of crisis in our lives. The sources of stress are all around us. Much of our behavior is a response to demands that come from many directions. Such demands range from the traumatic experiences to the subtle demands which frequently go unnoticed.

We are creatures of habit. Over a period of time we develop certain styles and routines that become deeply ingrained. Many are living life in the fast lane not because they have to but because they have developed the habit of a certain life-style.

Our rushing around and overextended ways are frequently reinforced by the attention and approval of other people. Stress becomes a way of life and our bodies remain in a constant state of readiness. We may not be sure what we are ready for; we just know we are geared up for something. Stress becomes the norm, whether legitimately or not. The clock strikes five o'clock. We foolishly think we can shift gears and by the time we reach home be totally relaxed. There is a tendency of the body to perpetuate a stress response.

My family operates two vehicles. One has an automatic transmission and the other has a manual shift. I personally have some difficulty changing from one car to the other. After driving the manual shift and then changing to the automatic, I will for a period of time continue to press the floorboard, looking for the clutch. Then after changing back to the manual shift, I will occasionally stop the car and forget to press the clutch. Why? We are creatures of habit. Our bodies seek constancy and resist the need to change.

Think how ironic and unreasonable it is to think that we are to work and remain at a certain level of activity with our nervous systems functioning in such a way and then, all of a sudden, at 5:00 PM or on Saturday morning we are not going to do that any more.

The body is a very smart and discriminative organism. The body senses what level of activity within what context it must perform and establishes a regulator called homeostasis. The body is a homeostatic mechanism that is both brilliant and ironically stupid at the same time. Once homeostasis is established, there is some difficulty in changing to a different level of functioning.

With the body set at this level of functioning, we think all this is supposed to change immediately without ever learning an active relaxation response. Rest is not inactivity. Rest is an active response whereby we become aware of the demands placed upon us and consciously seek to change our level of functioning to correspond to different surroundings. To effectively bring this into being, one must call upon mental, emotional, physiological, and spiritual capacities. Otherwise, the body may remain in high gear during times that could be used for revitalization. Rest is an active discipline.

In order to understand stress, we must first look at some basic ways in which the human body works. The body is an absolutely fascinating organism with a variety of parts and chemical substances. Changes are constantly occurring as one moves through the normal routines of daily living. The changes of the body, however, must be kept within limits. The internal environment of our bodies must maintain a degree of consistency. Blood pressure constantly changes to meet the demands placed upon the body. Heart rate, oxygen level, and other chemicals within the blood change to meet those demands. If any one function changes too much, the body cannot take it and the ultimate phase is death.

The demands that are placed upon the body can be outside agents, such as injury, germs, threats, or any one of thousands of emergency situations. The body is amazing in its ability to make adjustments when any change threatens to go too far. The body is an adaptive organism with a built-in desire to survive and does so by attempting to adapt and adjust as demands are experienced.

The most recognizable demands are the obvious threats of danger. Consider the young boy playing in a Little League baseball game who is running with all of his strength to catch an outfield fly ball only to collide with another boy stretching for the same ball. Upon impact many changes begin to take place within the child's body. The paleness reflects the shifts in circulation that makes sure his heart and brain will get enough blood. His panting keeps up his oxygen levels. His clotting mechanisms were readied to reduce his loss of blood. A tremendous number of changes are taking place as the body adapts to the threat from without.

Consider also the reaction of the father who is sitting on the second row of the bleachers. He is no stranger right now to stress. As he views the violent impact, his body begins immediately to adapt to a threat that is both without and within. His blood pressure changes, heart rate increases, adrenaline pours into his bloodstream, and his body gears up for an adaptive response to the threatening circumstances of his son. He not only quickly moves toward his son who is lying on the ground but also hurdles a chain link fence which on any normal occasion he could not have jumped.

After this emergency alarm reaction, many other responses go on much longer and represent the body's general response to a threat of any type. In the case of the boy and his father, changes occur all over the body to mobilize its defenses and protect it against harm. No one could question the impact of such emergency situation upon someone. The threat occurs and we react. We are adaptive creatures by nature.

Stress is also an issue in the long-term demands that are placed upon the body. Many professions are very stressful. There may be domestic problems at home which take years or even a lifetime to solve. The body is just as involved in long-term threats as in those acute, emergency situations. Even when we have for the moment forgotten our problems, stress may continue within our bodies. Stress is our body's reaction to any threat, real or imagined. From a practical standpoint our bodies windup faster than they wind down. Just because the clock indicates 5:00 PM and our calendar says vacation time has begun, our bodies do not take on a leisure-like style quite so suddenly. In fact, indications of stress continue well into the time when we feel that we should be relaxed.

A certain amount of anxiety may result from not being

able to settle down during a period of time when we are supposed to be relaxing. Because of the pace and stress of most life-styles our bodies usually are several days behind. We may be experiencing Sunday and are supposed to be resting but our bodies are still geared up for Friday's routine.

I have discovered that on vacation trips I am halfway through the week, if I am lucky, before I can settle down and become the lazy beach bum I inwardly long to be. Most of us are so geared toward production that considerable adjustment is necessary physiologically, emotionally, mentally, and spiritually before we can be at peace with our need for rest. We can rest more effectively if we have a better understanding of stress and how it affects us, whether we are aware of that effect or not. Much of our understanding of stress is rather recent.

The term *stress* was coined by Hans Selye, a professor at the University of Montreal. He wrote a classic book on stress, *The Stress of Life*, and used as a base for his writings an impressive number of medical research findings. Most of the studies described the bodily reaction to just about every conceivable type of demand. Selye noticed that certain features were common to all of them. In addition to specific changes, such as the rash of measles, the bruise of an injury, some nonspecific reactions were found in all and to these he gave the name *stress*. Selye noted that stress response was generalized and adaptive. Changes occur as a result of the body's attempt to mobilize defense against damage.

Therefore, stress occurs when one is awakened in the night by a sudden noise in the house. The body mobilizes for fight or flight. Yet, the stress response is just as real when the daily pressures of the job begin to get under our skin. Both sets of circumstances generate a stress response within the body.

Selye noted that the central role is played by the two tiny adrenal glands. While the inside part of the glands manufactures adrenaline, the outer layer produces two other types of important hormones. One regulates the amount and distribution of body fluids and their dissolved mineral salts and helps to maintain blood pressure. The other hormones build up stores of energy-supplying sugars. These hormones also influence certain antiinflammatory effects and help the body cope with potential infection.

Some physicians now feel that Selye overemphasized the role of the adrenals because several other glands play an important part in gearing up the body for a potential threat. Selye's contribution to the study of stress is undeniable as he points to the wisdom of the body in a stress response.

One point needs to be made very clearly. The tendency is to think of stress as an enemy. Stress, on the other hand, is not only normal to our daily routine but also vital. Without it we could not live very long. Man has survived through the ages because of this mechanism. So much of what physicians do is to remove the interferences so that our body and its natural defense mechanisms can work according to design.

Dr. Hans Selye was not the first person to take note of the body's reaction to danger. Dr. David H. Fink wrote in the early 1940s, in *Release from Nervous Tension,* concerning the role of the interbrain, later to be called the hypothalamus. When the interbrain senses a threatening situation, mechanisms are thrown into gear to start up what Fink referred to as a fear response.

Fink tried to restrict the usage of the word *fear* to refer to a compound of physical and mental processes rather than fear being an emotional experience. He hoped to equate fear with what we do with our entire body in response to danger. The stages Fink cataloged in a fear response were amazingly similar to the observations of Selye. First, we perceive a threat. Second, we desire to escape that danger. Third, certain bodily responses follow the intellectual process. Fourth, some of the bodily responses stir up disagreeable sensations which we seek to eliminate. And fifth, we seek to find relief in safety. If we cannot find safety, feelings may become so intense as to produce a paralyzing state.

While Selye's observations were much more accurate and precise, Fink also pointed to the fact that a price is required for anyone under stress. Stress, fear according to Fink, creates both a need for routine, preventive maintenance, and a physiological process that can inhibit the very thing, rest, which is needed for revitalization and recovery.

Selye would differ with Fink who theorized that the combinations of organ behavior are too many to be counted. Danger may bring about an infinite number of bodily organ combinations which constitute one's emotional range. Selye simplified the process by theorizing that the body's response to danger is essentially the same in all circumstances. Some simply carry the process further, and some are greater in intensity. Therefore, stress is stress is stress.

The point is still obvious; a cost is involved in the body's response to one's environment. This response creates both the need for rehabilitative rest as well as a physiological process which interferes with rest.

Some of our confusion about the role of stress has come from a basic misunderstanding of what is meant by the word *stress*. Stress is not an event that happens to us but is, instead, our body's response to the event. In the case of the father who observed his son's collision the stress was not the son's impact. The stress was the father's bodily response to the son's accident. For the son the stress was not the impact but his body's response to the experience. In the case of a demanding job, the stress is not the pressures of the work but the response one makes to the demands that are being experienced.

Stress is not always negative. Stress can be experienced in very positive ways, even ordinary events. Stress occurs when one proudly runs in a local race held for some charity. Stress is experienced by one who inherits a large sum of money. Stress can result even in a job one thoroughly enjoys. Severe stress is frequently a health factor for one who has achieved success in one's profession. Notoriety, for example, may become an extremely stressful situation.

Stress is not an experience of nervous anxiety but rather a state or condition of the body in response to a demand. Regardless of the demand, the body's response is still called stress. Hans Selye has described three stages in the body's adaptation response to a stressor (the agent making the demand).

The first stage is the alarm reaction. When a stressor is recognized, consciously or subconsciously, the brain sends a message to the pituitary gland, a small gland at the base of the brain, which secretes adrenocorticotrophic hormone (ACTH). When this hormone enters the bloodstream, the adrenal glands secrete adrenaline which then places the entire body on alert. Breathing rate increases along with heart rate and blood pressure. According to Dr. Joe Richardson,

The body thereby acts to provide oxygen-rich blood to

nourish the brain and the central nervous system, as well as the major muscle groups. Sugar stored in the body is dumped into the bloodstream to provide quick energy. Muscles tense and become coil-like to be ready to spring into action. The body perspires in order to cool itself during the increased activity. The pupils of the eyes dilate to allow more light to increase visual capabilities. All senses quicken. The body is prepared for fight or flight. Chemicals within the blood that facilitate rapid clotting are readied in case of an injury. Bodily processes not essential for either fight or flight are slowed or stopped altogether. Digestion slows or ceases so that blood is available for the brain and for major muscle groups. Bowel and bladder muscles relax to concentrate tension elsewhere in the body.[1]

Keep in mind that this response is generalized and non-specific and occurs in practically all experiences of stress. In other words, our general reaction to the pressure of work or even continued domestic problems is the same as when we are startled in the night by threatening noise.

The second stage is the resistance stage. This particular stage of the stress response is much slower than the alarm reaction which occurs quickly. If the stressor remains and if the body can accommodate the threat, the body moves into the more controlled resistance stage. Many threats are resolved quickly. The noise might be explainable. The ugly letter from the IRS was a mistake. The argument with our spouse was a misunderstanding. The car which stalls in traffic finally cranks again. Many stresses come and go. On the other hand, some stressors cannot be accommodated. Obviously, in a fatal automobile accident the body is not given a chance to go into the resistance phase.

During the resistance phase, the body seeks to adapt

and cope with the stressor. The endocrine system continues to produce hormones that activate the body's defenses. As the body adapts there are some obvious results.
One common, long-term effect is elevated blood pressure.
Over an extended period of time a number of diseases
associated with stress become likely. Stress is not the only
cause of coronary artery disease, ulcers, diarrhea, consti-
pation, backaches, headaches, and strokes; but stress may
be traced to be the source of many such problems. Stress
is often a confounding factor instead of a source. And do
not ignore the influence of stress on chemical dependency.

The third stage occurs when the stressors are severe
and become unmanageable. If the body is required to
maintain itself in this resistance stage long enough, the
body will lose its adaptive ability. The glands and muscles
simply cannot exist forever in the fight or flight dilemma.
Most of us take steps before or, at least, as we begin to
reach this stage. Our headaches, digestive problems, or
other symptoms usually force us to deal with our stress. By
now the point should be obvious. Our poor ways of dealing with the stress in our lives very drastically affects the
quality of our rest. One simply cannot spend eight to
twelve hours under tremendous pressure at work and
expect to walk in the back door at six o'clock, lay coat and
brief case in the chair, and become a model of relaxation.
If you can change gears that quickly, you are in a minority!

Stress is not inherently bad. Many of us do our best work
when under stress. We not only produce more, but there
is a certain feeling of exhilaration that goes along with a
managed, optimal level of stress. To remove stress from
our life would be a ludicrous goal. Our goal should be to
keep our stress at an optimal level.

An oversimplified comparison might be made to an automobile engine. A certain amount of tension and heat is needed for the engine to operate at peak performance. Most of us know how sluggish an engine can be before it warms up. On the other hand, under too much strain and heat the engine will definitely break down. Our bodies require a similar balance. An optimal level of stress is desirable for us to operate efficiently. Let the stress become too great for too long and we will break down. While some persons appear to adapt more readily than others, all of us have our limits.

The management of stress is far too complicated to go into great detail here. However, there are a few simple techniques we can develop which will not only help us relax and rest but also help us to possibly concentrate on some pressing matter of the moment. Numerous suggestions could be made at this point. As they relate to rest, allow me to mention only four.

A simple breathing exercise can do wonders. A rhythmical deep breathing pattern can relax the entire body. Usually as we fall asleep, we begin to breathe slower, deeper, and more relaxed. As our body becomes warm and relaxed, sleep becomes our gentle friend. Yet, why waste this restful pleasure in only the sleep state?

Find a restful place and get comfortable. Loosen any tight clothing that might inhibit circulation. Settle back and close your eyes. Let your body relax to the best of your ability. Take a deep breath and exhale. Take another, and release the breath with a sigh. Concentrate totally on your breathing, and become very aware of the air entering and leaving your body. Inhale through your nose, and exhale through your mouth. Notice the rhythm of your breathing. Breathing is a part of the rhythm of life. With each breath you take, become aware of the tension in your body. But, continue to concentrate upon your breathing. Notice the warmth that is permeating your body from the oxygen that is flooding your system. Notice the heaviness of your body as you continue to breathe. This rhythmical deep-breathing pattern is an excellent way to bring the body to a restful state.

A second strategy can be closely related to the first. Some of us may have difficulty with relaxation because we do not know what the state feels like. This simple discipline can be an exercise as well as a process of informing us. Other names may be given to the process such as biofeedback and stress release. We can actually relax by creating muscle tension. In a restful position, and after some deep-breathing exercises, begin to concentrate on the various parts of your body. Beginning with the extremities of feet and hands concentrate on specific muscles. Think of only one muscle at a time. As you concentrate on a single specific muscle, tense that muscle and release the tension. Thinking only of that muscle notice the contrast between the tense state and relaxed state. Tense and relax that muscle several times, and continue to notice the contrast. After working on that muscle for a moment, move to another and concentrate totally on it. Work your way in from the feet and hands and then give attention to the larger muscles of the back, stomach, and neck. Even your face has muscles that can be tensed and relaxed. You can take as long for this exercise as time permits. This can be used as a way to fall asleep.

A third suggestion related to dealing with stress has to do with exercise. While our culture has become increasingly aware of the need for exercise, we continue to be overweight and underexercised. A good exercise program is not limited to the guy who runs twenty miles a week. Jogging may be a part of your program, but it is certainly not the only way to exercise. A fast walk that provides twenty minutes of aerobic exercise four times a week is worth its weight in gold. The options for exercise are endless. They are beneficial only if appropriate and maintained. If tennis is your game, great. But, remember that all the tennis paraphernalia sold in all the stores in town is no substitute for getting out and playing the game. I have known some people who have a closet full of jogging shoes and have spent lots of money on all the electronic devices that are available but never get around to running. The exercise of removing one's wallet and buying all the gear is not an aerobic exercise.

The reason exercise is so important is obvious. Stress is a generalized response. The body is all geared up to do something and frequently there is nothing to which all the energy and force may be applied. Exercise provides a specific activity to which the body can respond. Race an automobile engine in neutral long enough and hard enough and a breakdown is inevitable. Not only are we providing a channel for our stress to be released but also we can use our stress to do some things that bring joy and excitement.

A fourth suggestion in dealing with stress is so obvious that it seems trite to mention. We cannot ignore the role of our diet in dealing with stress, as well as learning to rest. Remember that stress extracts a price. As the body adapts to a threat many chemical changes take place. Oxygen increases as the heart beats faster, blood pressure increases, muscles are provided with oxygen-rich blood, and blood sugar provides energy for adaptive measures. Energy resources must be provided for our body to function well under normal daily stresses as well as moments of emergency.

Dr. Joe Richardson offered seven suggestions that will help us manage stress:

1. Decrease intake of salty food. Sodium tends to increase blood pressure.
2. Decrease intake of junk food. Sweet or salty foods are not beneficial. Recent research has indicated reduced performance following sugar intakes because of the large increase in insulin.
3. Decrease intake of caffeine. Caffeine is a stimulant and raises the body's adrenaline level. Also, avoid products associated with nicotine.
4. Decrease intake of cholesterol-rich food. Cholesterol reduces the oxygen-carrying ability of the blood by reducing the diameter of blood vessels.
5. Increase intake of fresh fruit and vegetables. Vitamins and minerals of fruit and vegetables are vital to the adaptive processes of the body. For example, vitamin C which is found in fruit is depleted in the body by adrenaline and must be replaced.
6. Increase intake of whole grains. Magnesium which plays a role in relaxing muscles and regulating the heartbeat is found in whole grains. Also, fiber is a beneficial element in regulating bowel habits that are victimized by stress.
7. Increase intake of milk products. Calcium plays a role in reducing blood pressure. However, to avoid cholesterol one should purchase low-fat products.[2]

The relation of stress and rest is obvious. On one hand, rest is one of those precious ways of managing stress, a way to maintain that optimal level of stress that results in peak performance. On the other hand, unmanaged stress can become a severe deterrent to the process of rest. Rest and stress are not enemies. They are partners in the process of making us productive persons.

Notes

1. Joe Richardson, "The Christian and Stress" (Nashville: The Sunday School Board of the Southern Baptist Convention, 1975), p. 6.

2. Ibid., p. 27.

11

Time Management and Rest

"How can one possibily find rest when a cloud of unfinished business constantly hangs over one's head! There is so much to do, and most of the demands are really important. In fact, most of them are from home and work. How do you say no without feeling like a jerk?"

People who value their existence will try to make a contribution to their surroundings. However, for the average person this contribution does not come in the form of one single profound experience. Most of us make contributions by giving of ourselves through a multiplicity of demands. And to be honest, most of these demands are not in the form of earth-shattering experiences. They come in the form of the endless responsibilities of daily life. These routine, but important, demands take an unlimited number of forms and come at us from every direction.

One of life's great inhibitors of genuine rest is the anxiety of unfinished business. How do you rest in the evening when at quitting time there still seems to be more to do than when you began in the morning? This problem may be particularly familiar to the professional person who functions without a rigid checklist or specific time frames. Such a problem may be just as familiar to the housewife who has more to do and more places to go than she can possibly complete.

Time pressures are an inevitable part of modern life, and consequently, an acceptable level of personal productivity partially depends on wise management of our time. To even a casual observer the appearance is that the tempo and complexity of our routine life-styles is on the increase. We have to pack within days, and sometimes hours, the work that formerly took weeks or months. Yet, one reason some of us become overwhelmed by the demands placed on us is that we are terribly poor managers of our time. Poor time management inevitably leads to anxiety, frustration, and, occasionally, full-blown anger, which certainly works against effective rest.

One premise must be clearly understood. Time is a limited commodity. Many of us manage time as if it were an unlimited resource. The one who said "time has no beginning and no end" did not have to work, raise a family, go to church, and "chair" the PTA.

None of us would argue that a dollar can be spent only once. We might wish otherwise, but we know the truth. Time is a resource just like our money. Time can be spent only once. When it is gone, it is gone! Most of us live and manage our daily affairs as if time were an unlimited commodity. Much of our anxiety and wretched restlessness comes from trying to spend our time more than once. Time can be stretched but not reused.

The only way to avoid such anxiety is to make good decisions about how our time is to be spent. To improve our stewardship of time, we must first claim responsibility for ourselves and we must assume the role of a manager of time instead of a victim of time.

Do not forget that when faced with increasing demands on our time, we do have some choices. One option is to pass up the challenge of time and to accept less by default. To state it in terms of production, we can just produce a lot less than is our capability and learn to live with the results. If demands are getting to us, one has the option to make only one change. Cut back on production expectation and leave everything else as is, which is a rather poor option.

Second, we can go at it harder and give it more energy. If we are involved in routine panic eight hours a day, increase it to twelve. If we have a rugged constitution, we may do relatively well for a while under this growing burden, but we do have our limits. We may, however, discover fewer and fewer people wanting to draw near to us as we proceed because we will grow increasingly weary and insensitive. Another fact to consider is our diminishing ability as pressure builds and our judgment becomes more and more distorted by stress.

A third choice is to ignore one's habits altogether. We can take a victim's stance and assume that the problem lies with an overdemanding world. A clue that this is happening may be our narrowing ability to see only the trees at the expense of the forest. Our skin becomes quite thin as our emotional antennae stretch to the limit. Our attitudes toward our personal colleagues becomes increasingly critical as we make endless excuses for ourselves.

These choices offer very little promise of positive change. None of them solve the problem of time pressures. To shift from a passive to an active role and to change from a victim's outlook to a manager's perspective requires significant self-analysis. If one is not willing to face up to ineffective ways of managing time, personal improvement is just a pipe dream. One must make deliberate effort to do things differently.

The results of this positive change will be twofold. First, one's personal productivity will increase. Who of us would not like to be more productive? Second, increased control will mean less frustration and anxiety. Honest efforts to manage time more effectively will have a significant impact on one's ability to rest.

The word *deliberate* must be used in regard to time management. The reason is obvious. In order to improve one's stewardship of time a determined and deliberate effort must be made. A casual, incidental approach to better time management will seldom produce results. Victor Hugo once said, "When the disposal of time is left to the chance of incidence, chaos will reign."

Many of our problems come from bad and ineffective habits. And habits are not easily changed. Consider just how many of our daily activities are performed out of habit. We shave, dress, eat, drive to the office, and do many of the routine functions of our work as a matter of habit. The result is that our attention is somewhere else other than on the task at hand. Through habit we conduct most of our business. We eat, sleep, think, judge, and remember without being alert to what is going on. The bottom line is that we may be guilty of poor habits that are terribly ineffective and not even realize it. Habits can be changed only by conscious efforts.

Changing from a victim to a manager of time requires alertness. We must protect our freedom to manage our time, and poor habits become our freedom's greatest enemy. To do so is not to aim for a constant state of bug-eyed watchfulness. Habits relieve us from the exhaustive boredom of repetitive tasks. If not guarded, however, habits can take over the bulk of our controls and become less than a friend.

The number one culprit of poor time management is a lack of concentration. Alert concentration is a primary component of effective time usage. In moments, even hours, of preoccupation, the incidents are born which swallow up hours and days of precious time.

Consider a typical morning which just might be the experience of many of us. For days I have planned this Saturday morning to be the time when I would tend to an embarrassingly crowded attic. I have been dreading this chore and procrastinating for months. Saturday morning is here, and I am going to be task oriented.

Of course the day would begin better with a good breakfast. The smell of sausage will make even a dusty attic smell better. I check the refrigerator, and there is no sausage. The local grocery is not far away, and I can pick up some boxes for storage while I am there. I will be back in no time.

On my way I notice that the car is almost out of gas. They do run better with gas! The station is near and will require only a minute. The cars are lined up. Why is everybody wanting gas this time of morning? My turn finally comes, and I think I'll check the oil while I am here. The left front tire looks low to me. To get air now costs a quarter. What is the world coming to? I have no change. The guy in the window has plenty, and he will be glad to give me change. Now the quarter hangs in the slot.

The operator notices and says that he'll be right over to retrieve my money. He gets the air going, and I can tend to my tire. The gas pump works, and I am in business. As I drive out of the station, I realize I forgot to pay for the gas. They frown on nonpayment and jail is not in my plans for today!

Finally, I am at the grocery store, along with everyone else north of the Mexican border. The sausage cooler has twenty-three different kinds, and I notice that some of the packages note that their product has less cholesterol. I read the labels of a few, pick one, and make my way to the cashier. My wife has the check-cashing card, so I have to get out of line and go to the service desk. Evidently lots of other people need the same thing. Finally, I'm on my way home with the sausage.

Breakfast was really nice. Since the weather was so good we ate outside at the patio table. One more cup of coffee, a quick look at the paper, and I will be attic-bound. No one has picked up the paper, so I make my way to the box by the street. On the way I notice the shrubs by the door look terribly dry. We have not had any rain in six weeks. As you might guess, Bill, who lives next door, borrowed the hose. Since his wife has been sick lately, this will give me a good reason to check on her.

The shrubs are watered and while I am doing this I might as well hook up the sprinklers and water the lawn. Everything looks so dry. Now for the paper. Where is it? I left it next door at Bill's. When I knock on the door Bill already is bringing the paper to the door for me. "While you are here, would you help me move the piano? We have finally decided to move it out of the living room." We move the piano.

Back at the house I settle down with my cup of coffee, which my wife has warmed three times already. She informs me that while she was warming it, she noticed that the cat has chewed the insulation off the cord on the microwave. Until I can get it to the service shop, I had better wrap some tape around the wire.

On the way to the attic, I hear the familiar sounds of the garbage truck. None of the house cans have been emptied, and the main one is not by the road. The garbage truck backfires and rolls to the curb and when the driver sees me bringing my trash to the street, he asks if I would call the office and let them know that the truck has broken down. Of course, I would.

The morning is getting late as I notice the mail truck go by. One quick check and I'll be ready to go to work. One of the letters is the heating repair bill which indicates that I did not make last month's payment. They are wrong! I have the cancelled check to prove it. They are in the desk drawer, I think. I had better check to see if I have a right to get mad. The check is there; so I'll call the central office. They put me on hold. Since it is Saturday, they do not have many representatives working. The matter is cleared. The reason was easy. The payment missed the computer deadline by one day. Everything was fine.

As I make my way to the attic, my wife informs me that lunch is ready and that after lunch we must go to the reception which we had discussed. The attic never did get cleaned and, for all practical purposes, the day was spent and also wasted.

The story might be a little extreme but very close to home for many of us. Not only is there the frustration of not accomplishing the task but now there is the aggravation of having to plan it again when, in fact, next Saturday needs to be donated to the PTA project. A little thing, yes, but still quite frustrating and a source of restless aggravation.

The problem was simple and obvious. There was no concentration on the task. Preoccupation turned this soul into a victim of the day instead of a manager of the day.

Poor concentration may be found as a dynamic of practically every wasted day.

Instead of concentrating on the task at hand, which was cleaning the attic, everything was allowed to interrupt and demand attention. In other words, get up, eat breakfast with or without sausage, and get busy with the attic. Preoccupation is a thief when we value our time.

I am not saying that one should become obsessively compulsive. But, if cleaning the attic is the goal for the morning, get with it! The chances are good that cleaning the attic really is not a very exciting task and, therefore, it does not take much to distract. Frustration and restlessness for most people in regard to time can usually be measured by the frequency of interruptions. The poorest management of time occurs in the daily routine events. Consider your network of routines. Remember, we are creatures of habit. You have your routine of walking, dressing, eating, going to work, numerous routines at work, and the way you bring your day to a close. There are also routines for socializing, church, and cutting the grass. This is not to imply for a moment that you should not have routines. The problem is that during these habits of behavior your preoccupation and lack of concentration is at peak levels.

Alertness is down. Preoccupation is up. And one becomes a victim to poorly used time. Possibly you have always bought groceries on Saturday morning. So does practically everyone else. Be alert and consider the possibility of buying groceries on Tuesday afternoon when the store is practically empty.

The key is simple. Take note of how you spend your time, when you spend your time, and where you spend your time. Observation of one's own behavior can be quite revealing. Yet, very few people make the effort to evaluate the way they spend their most valuable resource, time.

Let me pass along some very elementary suggestions that might be of help. The first suggestion has already been stated. Observe what you do with your time. Do not be a victim to habit. If you are uncomfortable with your routine or especially if you feel trapped by constant demands, stop and take an honest mental assessment of yourself.

Second, assign some labels to your time. Divide a normal week into parts. Try to attach some labels to the parts which might identify the way that part is spent. Take note if there is a sense of balance to your time.

Let me give you an example of the way a business colleague of mine has identified his professional time. He places all his time into one of four categories: (1) pay-off time, (2) investment time, (3) organizational time, and (4) wasted time. When on the job, he must label all his time in one of the four categories. The key for him is to make sure there is a sense of balance. For example, pay-off time is the time spent in the bringing of a business deal to a close. That kind of experience would never take place without having spent investment time previously in making it come about. Organizational time is spent making the refinements and adjustments in the system which continually needs attention and brings no immediate tangible results. Everything that does not fall into one of these three categories for this good man falls into wasted time.

Now, keep in mind that this man's self-observation is strictly for his business life but the point should be clear. You may find no interest at all in dividing your time up into such categories. Make up your own and discover if there is a sense of balance to your expenditure of time.

Let me give you a very simple example of a young man

who is a sales representative. He is, first, an individual with appropriate time demands and needs. Second, he is also a married man with appropriate time demands and needs. Third, he is also a businessman with appropriate time demands and needs. Fourth, he is also a parent with appropriate time demands and needs. Fifth, he is active in his church with appropriate time demand and needs. Most of his time can be thrown into these categories. Each part is important and worthy. Trouble occurs when one or two categories account for practically all of his time.

Let me offer a third suggestion. As you shift from victim to manager, learn to organize and prioritize. Plan your day. Make some goals for yourself as you organize your time. Consider the mundane tasks, as well as the larger responsibilities.

Make a list of what you hope to accomplish in a given day and establish some priorities. The best friend a good manager of time has is a piece of paper. Learn to make a list. A piece of paper can relieve your brain of a great amount of work. Your brain has enough to do already.

As you plan, make room for the routine duties and the larger responsibilities. Your plan and list should make room for both, and they should be at appropriate intervals. Take care of some of the mundane chores first, but do not allow yourself to become bogged down with only the mundane tasks.

At the end of the day, check your list and start another one for tomorrow. The entire process of planning and even making the lists help you to claim responsibility for yourself and your day. Such planning will also help to keep you on track. Unless you claim the right to manage your time, you will only respond to the outside world.

A fourth suggestion is that you periodically look at the big picture. Back away from the trees periodically and look at the forest. Just as you should organize and set goals for each day, consider what you plan for the next month. Working in the larger blocks of time will give some exciting flexibility while providing direction.

A fifth suggestion is that you plan some time for doing nothing. Everyone needs time to "be." There is little that makes us more ready for action than a brief period of inactivity. A friend of mine once told me that when he got to busy to lie on his living room floor and roll up lint balls, he was too busy. I am not suggesting that you should find some strange pleasure in lint balls, but my friend's point is good advice. We all need time to occasionally do nothing.

We usually rest well when we have worked hard. We rest even better when we feel like we have accomplished our tasks. To continuously leave tasks unfinished is a terrific source of unrest. We have all been there at some point in time.

The reasons for not meeting the demands placed on us are many. Over-commitment, poor preparation, and lack of ability are always possibilities. The chances are that poor time management is also a factor. God has granted us only so much time. When a minute is gone, it is gone forever. We cannot call it back. We are, therefore, to be good stewards of our time, just as we are to be good stewards of all of our resources. Such an attitude about time is our Christian duty. Such an attitude also makes good sense.

"To everything there is a season, A time for every purpose under heaven" (Eccl. 3:1).

12

The Sunday Rest,
an Unappreciated Gift

Generally speaking, our society is ignoring a very special gift. The observance of the sabbath is undeniably one of the most unclaimed blessings of the human experiment. From the beginning, the observance of the sabbath was to provide rest and revitalization after a demanding week.

The second chapter of Genesis describes with clarity the purpose of this seventh day. Holy Scripture indicates that after the heavens and earth were finished, God rested on the seventh after His work was done. God also sanctified this seventh day since on that day He had rested from His work. If work is to have a diminishing effect on body and spirit, provision must be made for the replenishing of those physical and spiritual energies. By sanctifying this day of rest God has therefore made provision for one of the most basic of human needs, rest.

As the Christian community came to observe the first day of the week, Sunday, as a time of rest, another dimension was added to the observance. The Christian church began celebrating the first day of the week in honor of the Lord's resurrection. Our sabbath was no longer just a day of physical restraint. The celebration and worship which followed the Lord's resurrection incorporated a much-needed spiritual dimension to rest. Sabbath, at its best, replenished both the physical and spiritual energies. To ignore such an opportunity borders on outright foolishness.

For all practical purposes our society has ignored the inherent benefits of God's provision. We are weaker because of it. A great need exists for us to reconsider the use of the sabbath, which for Christians is now Sunday. For all practical purposes the secular world ignores it, and the religious community varies from indifference to legalism.

The strict observance of the sabbath grew out of the traditions in Israel. Regardless of the exact time when the sabbath was first observed in Israel, the significance goes back to the story of creation. The establishment of a day of rest is not a result of human decision-making but the result of a divine ordinance. Holy Scripture makes quite clear the role of the sabbath in God's plan.

Sabbath keeping is an undisputable fact in the Bible. In other words, because the writer of Genesis included the sabbath as a part of the original constitution of nature, the universal application of sabbath rest applies to all people. The original observance goes beyond superficial practice. The twenty-third chapter of Exodus states emphatically that one's ox and colt must be given the opportunity for rest. The fifth chapter of Deuteronomy includes one's servants as having the right to sabbath rest.

As the synagogue became more important to early Israel, the sabbath came to be not only a day of rest but also a day of worship. Thus, this day of rest provided the opportunity for the refreshment of body and spirit.

As is the possibility with any observance, orthodoxy became the primary issue. The restrictions became so rigid that life became cramped within the system. The practice of the sabbath became so excessive that rest gave way to confinement. One was not free to rest but, instead, one was cramped by the rigid restrictions. The observance was obviously carried too far when rabbis would debate whether a cripple were guilty if his house caught on fire on the sabbath and he had to carry out his wooden leg.

The observance of Sunday by the Christian community has at times reflected some of the same legalism of the Jewish sabbath. The Puritans of New England could easily have been "first cousins" to the first-century Jewish scribes and Pharisees. Much of what we are experiencing today as we ignore the Sunday traditions is a reaction to the excess of our Puritan forefathers.

The Puritans and their spiritual descendants have given many people just the excuse they needed to throw the baby out with the bath water. While not deserving the total blame for the overreaction, the Puritan heritage has a way of dividing people into two categories. On the one hand, you could be painfully religious. Without ever meeting a first-century Pharisee one can imagine the "wrinkled" demeanor of one so righteous. That is one category.

On the other hand, you could be wantonly sinful. That is the other category. And we are left in some doubt as to which is worse! The Puritans, in the process, were describing the basic nature and tone of the Christian life. The first-century Pharisees were wrong and Jesus exposed them for what they were, lifeless as sepulchers. Francis of Assisi was right when he said, "Sadness belongs to the devil and his angels, but we knowing what we know, and

believing what we believe, what can we do except re-
joice!" One scholar has wisely said, "The sad man is always
sinning."

In an effort to get away from the puritanical inflexibili-
ty, most people have disregarded the value of a day of rest
as God's gift to a tired humanity. Our generation has once
again gone from one extreme to another.

However, the original message of the sabbath is still the
same. One cannot work indefinitely. One not only needs
rest from labor but also an opportunity for fresh perspectives. The observance of the sabbath should be a time
when our inner spirit finds expression. Physical rest which
offers no opportunity for the revitalizing of one's spiritual
needs will fall short of the mark.

Jesus took such a practical and wise approach to the
sabbath. He assisted people in need, as well as using the
day as a time to refresh His own inner spirit. Notice,
however, that the source of His strength was found in His
customary presence in the synagogue on the sabbath. To
state this practice in another way, Jesus went to church.

In the second chapter of Mark, Jesus tried to readjust
our thinking about the sabbath. Man was not created to
be a slave of the sabbath. Instead, the sabbath was created
for the benefit of all people. Within such a concept is
found a point that needs to be offered to our present
generation.

Men and women need to free themselves from the
need to do on Sunday whatever the old Sabbatarianism
restricted. We need to keep in mind the purpose of the
sabbath and take that purpose to full expression. The sabbath is for mankind's advantage, but not to ignore and
lose. It should be a day when, as for our Lord, we seek to
restore both the physical and spiritual energies that have
been depleted by the demands of the previous week.

As mentioned earlier, Sunday should provide an even more important role than could the seventh-day sabbath. Since the day of rest was shifted to the first day of the week to honor the resurrection of the Lord, Sunday should be a time for men and women to be raised from the rudimentary physical and spiritual concerns. Sunday can be a time of moving from the cold earth to the warmth of the light.

The way a gift is received is just as important as the way it is given. A gift may be offered with the wisest of intentions. Unless the recipient has enough wisdom to claim a gift, very little can be accomplished. God's sanctifying of the sabbath is more than ancient history. In so doing He has offered to each one of us a gift that has more power to redeem than most of us dare to realize. God blessed the seventh day and made it sacred in itself, but He also offers it to us as a source of well-being. If we disregard it or abuse it, we are the losers in the process.

Why have we disregarded such a precious gift? One reason has already been confessed. We possess a natural tendency to overreact. We may reject the puritanical straightjacket and, in so doing, we go to the other extreme and lose sight of the gift altogether. To ignore the sabbath is just as ridiculous as turning it into a prison sentence.

A second reason for our disregard is that many of us have relinquished the control of Sunday. We assume the role of the victim, a passive approach to Sunday. After all, if we claim no control and responsibility for the other six days why should we expect to claim control over Sunday? The use of Sunday is, once again, a matter of time management. If one envisions oneself as a victim of time, Sunday will be just another day of being kicked around.

A third reason for our disregard is our pushing for production beyond the level of good common sense. We make a foolish assumption that if a certain amount can be produced in six days we can produce more by adding the seventh day. The foolishness can be found in the disregard for routine maintenance. The finest of equipment must be periodically idle for repair. Maintain properly a quality automobile and one can expect years of dependable service. Buy the most expensive car on the road, drive it hard enough and long enough without idle time and maintenance, and the engine will soon disintegrate.

Why do almost all stores open on Sunday now? Two reasons. First, obviously, some of us had rather shop than rest. Second, if business can get so much of our money in six days, they can bleed us even more on a seventh day. The sad part of the story is that we do not even realize what we are doing to ourselves. We are caught in a vicious cycle of trying to produce more and more on less and less.

God has placed before us a precious gift. The sabbath was made for us that we might restore those physical, mental, emotional, and spiritual energies that have been pulled from us as we have sought to carry out our duties. Instead of being a wise steward of that gift, we have turned it into another demand that extracts yet more of life's vital energy.

Are you tired? Then consider how you spend your Sundays. Rest and worship can provide a powerful combination punch toward a demanding week which follows.

13

"Ultimate" Trust, the Real Issue

Rest is a very natural part of life, as natural as breathing out and breathing in. Yet we must not assume that rest occurs only when there is an absence of physical activity. Rest is much, much more. Any of us can recall a night of rolling and tossing. In theory we were lying down, but rest was not the result.

True rest involves the cooperation of all our capacities. There obviously must be periods of time when we are still and inactive. Adequate time must be allowed for our bodies to restore the vitality diminished by our work. No one can work indefinitely without granting time for these physical needs. Ignore these demands and our physiological system will eventually fail, regardless of one's constitutional strength. However, physical inactivity is only a part of the process.

We must also recognize the role of our emotions. The ability to understand and control one's emotions is a vital part of the resting process. The ability to feel separates us from all other creatures. Claiming our emotions primarily

means that we are not to be slaves to them. One who is
subject to the emotions of the moment can know little
peace.

Mental discipline must also be exercised if rest is to
occur. We are endowed with the mental capacity necessary to be responsible for ourselves. We do not have to be
rigid and compulsive to experience a well-ordered life.
Through the power of the mind we can control much that
happens without and within. A lack of concentration is a
frequent prelude to restlessness. To ignore our mental
capacities is to become physically irresponsible and emotionally immature.

As important as these capacities are, physical, emotional, and mental discipline are not enough. Something else
is needed to take up where our capacities end. Even the
most responsible person must live in the midst of many
variables over which one has little control. Given our
limited abilities we can only do so much to make everything work out favorably. Precisely at this point we must
recognize the most crucial dimension of rest. Genuine
rest requires a value system that goes beyond human
capacity. Life is composed of too many variables; and, if
circumstances are totally dependent upon our solitary
efforts, restlessness is inevitable.

Augustine's philosophy was, "There is no rest until we
find rest in Him." Such a description of rest is more than
just a nice sounding cliche. We must have something
beyond our own capacities if rest is to be complete.

The writer of Deuteronomy said, "The eternal God is
your refuge, And underneath are the everlasting arms"
(Deut. 33:27). Adeline Whitney, over a century ago, wrote
in response to that verse,

"The everlasting arms." I think of that whenever rest is

sweet. . . . No thought of God is closer than that. No human tenderness of patience is greater than that which gathers in its arms a little child, and holds it, heedless of weariness. And He fills the great earth, and all upon it, with this unseen force of His love, that never forgets or exhausts itself, so that everywhere we may lie down in His bosom, and be comforted.

The real issue at hand is that of trust, ultimate trust in the God of creation. Trust is not only one of the most significant issues of our faith but is also the very issue upon which our peace of mind depends.

Do you really trust God? Note that I did not ask if you could sing the old hymns about trust or if you could speak the religious language. Do you really trust God? Do you sincerely believe that God is a living, powerful reality? Do you believe that He is actively involved in the affairs of persons? Do you honestly feel that God takes pleasure in your joy, is actively seeking your happiness, and wants nothing more than to experience a smile on your face? Your response to these questions is undeniably one of the most significant and determining factors in your rest.

Trust has always been an issue. How better can you describe the problem of Adam and Eve in the Genesis account than that of mistrust? The inability to trust is precisely what turned a happy experience into a sad one.

Consider the setting. God placed Adam and Eve in the Garden of Eden and essentially instructed them to enjoy life and trust in Him. Obviously God had their best interests in mind or He would never have given them access to such joy. The one basic requirement was that they trust Him. Why shouldn't they trust Him? He certainly had given them no reason to do otherwise. Yet, apparently they began to have doubts about God's intention for them. Was His motivation really an attempt to keep them in their place? The thought must have been in their minds because they needed very little encouragement to offer a protest. We can try, if we choose, to blame the serpent, point to Eve, or use any number of excuses; but if man had trusted God's intentions, the outcome would have been totally different. Man did not trust God and, therefore, knocked over his own table in order to get to God's.

Since that time very little has changed. We talk about our trust in God's goodness but, for all practical purposes, most of us do not operate out of such a framework. We quickly quote from Romans 8:28 that God is at work for good in our lives and, yet, conduct our affairs as if the outcome of the world is totally upon our shoulders. We must claim our responsibilities but remember all the while that we are partners in the business and not sole owners.

Unless there is an undergirding belief in God's power and goodness, we will assume all of the responsibility for the outcome of events which surround us. When we do that, we are destined for weariness. Anxiety and restlessness is the inevitable result of assuming the total responsibility for our circumstances.

So much of the complexity of our modern day is the result of the lack of a value and faith system that goes beyond our personal capacities. If everything is up to us, we must go to great extremes to cover all the bases. Our hurried life-styles are a perfect example. The problems of our fast paced life-style are much deeper than the fatigue of routine rush. Our complicated lives result from a materialistic approach to life which assumes that if one buys, borrows, or leases enough, he or she will feel secure. Security will never flow from such an approach. Security comes when we realize that God is our partner and is working to bring about "good."

Richard J. Foster in his classic book, *The Celebration of Discipline,* very accurately ascribed much of our inner restlessness to a lack of inward simplicity. He described three inner attitudes which may be developed and give freedom from a great deal of anxiety.

First, we should recognize that what we have is a gift from God. The temptation is great and quite natural to assume that our possessions are a direct result of our hard work. Work is part and parcel to our human existence but the product of our labor can never be separated from the grace of God. An accident or misfortune very quickly reminds us how radically dependent we are on sources outside ourselves for everything. We are dependent upon God for our daily bread, whether we want to admit it or not.

Second, we should grant God the opportunity to care for what He has provided. God is more than capable of protecting what we seemingly possess. Once again, the issue is whether we actually trust God. One of the real growing edges in our spiritual maturity is learning to trust God with regard to material possessions. Does this mean that we should be negligent and unconcerned about inherent dangers? Of course not! Christian maturity is never to be sought at the expense of common sense. As Foster wisely stated, "Simplicity means the freedom to trust God for these (and all) things."[1]

The third inner attitude involves making our things available to other people. This attitude is quite difficult to develop because of our fear of the future. The temptation is great for us to cling to our possessions because of our anxiety about tomorrow. If we knew that after our goods were shared there would still be adequate resources for the future, our anxieties would be considerably less. To truly believe in God as the One who ultimately provides will encourage us to share because we know He will care for us. Once again, common sense should guide us as decisions are made about sharing. However, the point is obvious. Breaking our attachment to things frees us in many ways from restlessness.

The problem with trusting only in our own capacities is that more demand is placed on us than we can possibly meet. How can we ever do enough to keep all of life's control buttons under our own fingertips? Fatigue and frustration are the inevitable result of a solo act.

Much of our frustration as a culture comes from our relentless rushing. We are constantly running from one place to another, and usually we are so anxiously caught up in just getting from point A to point B that we are unaware of what is happening to us physically, emotionally, mentally, and spiritually.

There are times when we must get in a hurry. None of us totally control our circumstances so that we do not occasionally have to get with it. Yet a very high price is paid when rush becomes the primary characteristic of our life-style. Many of us have reached the point that if we are not out of breath, we feel guilty or possibly anxious that something is out of order. One psychologist has referred to our predominant cultural life-style as "routine panic."

In our rush we lose much of our discerning ability. Our perspectives become cloudy. In our frenzied pace we fail to achieve the very things we assume that will provide meaning for our lives even though we continue to seek them with intensified effort and increased anxiety. There is a great deal of sadness about our relentless rushing.

Dr. Reynolds W. Greene told the story of a young boy running down the street as fast as his legs would carry him, with a ticket clutched tightly in his hand. He could hear the music of the band as the circus carts of animals passed along the crowded streets. He reached his vantage point just as the elephants came by. The horses pranced by with the trapeze artists on their backs. For any child, young or old, circus parades are exciting. The last event in the parade was the clowns who were dressed in their usual bright costumes. The little boy reached into his pocket for his ticket, handed it to a clown, and turned to walk a mile and a half back to his house. The next day he learned too late that he had seen the parade but had missed the circus.

There is no humor to the story because it is a parable of many of our lives. We push ourselves in and out of many activities, most of which are very honorable. Yet we discover in retrospect that we have only experienced the parade and not the main show. The end result is frustration and frequently much misdirected anger. Frustration brings about anger, and the crisis for some may be found in deciding what to do with many strong, painful feelings.

Our frustration becomes a vicious cycle. The more we rush, especially without adequate rest, the less we are able to perceive accurately. We finally reach the point where we are not sure what is the parade and what is the circus. May our days be busy in the sense that they are filled with meaning. On the other hand, let us not equate meaning with frenzied activity. The unrelenting rush of today's life-style is not an indicator of the presence of meaning but rather its absence. The inevitable result of a solo act is very predictable.

The pressures of life are real and unrelenting. We determine in our hearts not to be ruled by them; but, at the end of each day, we continue to deal with our unwelcomed companions of fatigue and frustration. The spring in our step will come back only when we take a long and serious look at the way we transact our personal business.

Trust in regard to our faith is a relational issue, just as with other persons. In other words, trust operates best in the context of a personal relationship. Trust comes easier with persons we know well. Our trust level increases as we know God better. One way to help our cause is to take time to begin our day with God. To be conscious of our relationship to God at day's beginning will influence all the hours that follow. Evening time is too late to recognize that this is the day which the Lord has made and that we are to be glad in it. Such an awareness must begin with the day.

Most people today have no sense of rejoicing in their lives. Life means rush, not joy. Joy will never come unless we are willing to occasionally slow down between point A and point B. Joy will come when we clear our perception and increase our discerning abilities to experience the main event rather than settling for a parade. Joy will come when we let God rule in our lives and allow Him to direct our days instead of being directed by the pressures which constantly surround us.

If our day begins with an awareness of God's hand upon our shoulder so should the day proceed in an attitude of trust. One part of mature Christian stewardship is to give every day the best we have to offer and then learn how to trust God for the rest. Much of our need to rush comes from our efforts to control all of our circumstances. We can control only so much, whether we choose to admit it or not. The quality of our daily lives would be greatly enhanced if we would stop frantically rushing to seek solutions to all problems and learn how to "be still and know" that God is still God and that He is seeking our ultimate best. "There is no rest until we find rest in Him." Tolstoy called this searching a God-shaped blank within you which nothing else can fill.

Trusting within the context of our faith has a very practical value. Allow me to refer again to some very unusual research conducted in the sixties with some sheep. Experiments were conducted with sheep in a laboratory setting. The image of a square was placed before a sheep. If the sheep pressed a lever, food was given to the animal. If a circle was placed before the sheep and he pressed the lever, a mild shock was given to the animal. The sheep soon learned to tell the difference between the two images. At that point the researchers began shaving the corners off the squares so that more and more the squares began to resemble circles. Interestingly, the sheep who were being monitored began to exhibit serious signs of stress. The stress indication continued to increase as the squares looked more and more like circles. The shock being given to the sheep was not enough to justify the response of the animals since it was only strong enough to indicate a wrong response. The researchers concluded the increased stress response was due simply to the inability of the animals to distinguish squares from circles. Also significant was the fact that the animals did not completely recover from this experience. When they were placed back in the fields, they continued to exhibit abnormal behavior. They were much more easily frightened than animals not exposed to this experiment.

While caution must be exercised when interpreting the results of research with animals to the experiences of human beings, a theory becomes obvious. We need something in life to help us tell the difference between squares and circles. When we are unable to discern or distinguish, the result is anxiety and stress. A personal faith in which we can be confident can help us distinguish between the squares and circles facing us daily.

I am personally convinced that one of the reasons for

the increased anxiety level of people today is that many people have no value system outside their own feelings to guide them in the routine as well as the critical decisions of daily living. We must have something to help us distinguish squares from circles or restlessness is the inevitable result. A God in whom we trust does, indeed, have more than just a mystical application to our lives. A confident faith is a very practical matter that touches us at the roots of our existence.

One other point needs to be made. No person ever sank under the burden of the day. The weight becomes more than we can bear when tomorrow's problems are added to the problems of today. To load ourselves down in such a way makes little practical sense. If we find ourselves so loaded, we should remember that it is our own doing and not God's. Over and over again He has begged us to leave the future to Him and give our attention to the present.

Jesus said, "Do not worry about your life, what you will eat, or what you will drink; nor about your body, what you will put on" (Matt. 6:25). These words are good advice and they sound especially impressive when we offer them to someone else. Living by them is another story!

> One there lives whose guardian eye
> Guides our earthly destiny;
> One there lives, who, Lord of all,
> Keeps His children lest they fall;
> Pass we, then, in love and praise,
> Trusting Him through all our days,
> Free from doubt and faithless sorrow,
> God provideth for the morrow.
> —Reginald Heber

Note

1. Richard J. Foster, *The Celebration of Discipline* (New York: Harper and Row, 1978), p. 77

14

"Time Outs" and
Back into the Game

Mondays have always been tough. Getting back into the grind has never been an easy task. And then in the history of mankind came the one redeeming feature which saved Mondays, Monday night football. It's now Monday night and I am doing what every patriotic male, and some females, does, hanging on to every word of Mr. NFL himself, Frank Gifford. The game is close, with only fifty-five seconds left in the first half. Dallas has recovered a fumble on the Miami twenty yard line. Dallas is behind seven to three and a touchdown would send them into the dressing room at halftime with our fickle friend "Momentum" on their side.

The Dallas fans are screaming and Danny White does what any good quarterback should do, he calls a time-out. That time-out may be one of the most important offensive moves he will make all night. Dallas has not quit for the half. They have every intention of going back into the game with nothing less than a touchdown on their minds.

During the time out the players take a couple of needed

deep breaths, Danny White consults with Tom Landry, and everyone gets ready for a demanding series of plays. The whistle blows, White calls the play, and both lines are braced for the impact. Walker carries the ball around the right side, follows one block, sidesteps another Dolphin, and dives into the end zone. The old fickle friend "Mo" goes into the dressing room with the Cowboys.

The key to the success of this particular game was the wise use of a time-out. A time-out may be one way of stopping the clock, but its value far exceeds that purpose. In fact, a properly utilized time out may be one of the most strategic maneuvers in any timed athletic contest. In thinking more about this, I become interested in the thoughts of some who know the game well. What might they have to say about the use of a time-out?

University of Georgia coach Vince Dooley, one of the most highly regarded names in college football, had this to say about the use of time-outs:

> A time-out can, indeed, be more than a method of simply stopping the clock. Coaches consider time-outs invaluable strategic tools that are not to be wasted. They must be saved for crucial situations, especially when little time remains in the half or the game. They give coaches time to develop and relay strategy to the team in critical situations. A time-out can also be used to stop an opponent's momentum and give the team a chance to regain their breath. In many cases time-outs are called because of substitution problems and confusion on the field or even to avoid certain penalties.

Coach Phil Jones, a respected high school coach in Georgia, said:

> Time-outs are called because strategically the opposing team is being able to take advantage of some aspect of

your team's play. A time-out is called in an attempt to correct that situation prior to the opposing team taking full advantage. Time-outs are called in crucial situations to have the opportunity for your coaches to discuss a crucial situation and determine the best possible decision at the moment. Time-outs are called late in the half or game to stop the clock and conserve energy in order to score.

I personally found it very difficult to listen to the responses of these good men and not make all kinds of comparisons to life in general and, more specifically, to the role of rest as we play our game. Notice a very simple and obvious truth. A time-out is never to be envisioned as the end of the game. In other words, the plan is always to get back into the game and deal with the challenge at hand. A time-out always stops the clock; but when one is called, the clock is never unplugged and put away. The clock is only stopped temporarily. No one ever calls a time-out and then goes directly into the dressing room. The time-out is a means to an end, winning the game.

Such is the case with rest. Rest is not an end in itself. Rest is a time out with the purpose of getting back into the game. Rest is a sweet gift, a right, and to a degree, a reward, but it is never an end in itself. Rest is a means of remaining productive and performing more efficiently in the position to which each of us has been called. Such an understanding does not take away the sweetness of rest, but rather gives meaning to the process.

Do not be confused that I am assuming everyone is to be eternally employed from eight to five to be productive. One's particular role of productivity in life can take many forms. Neither does this position assume that rest is not a valid part of the retirement years. Retirement is an earned privilege, but productivity should continue right along. While the results of that productivity may not be measured by a regular paycheck, the opportunities to contribute to one's surroundings are always present.

Allow me to give an example. I have discovered that some of the wisest and most courageous people I know live in nursing homes. I was visiting recently with one dear lady who has just recently made the adjustment of the move from her personal home to a nursing facility. Her routine has dramatically changed in recent years, and rest consumes a greater percentage of her time now. But, as she rests, she is anticipating her afternoon walk down the hall. She will visit and share her God-given smile with the people whom she passes. The challenges of her life now are considerably different than they were ten years ago, but they are the tasks before her now. She is resting more now, but not because she has dropped out of the game. She is just playing a different position, and rest is her way of playing the game well.

On the other hand, I can recall another visit recently with a man who has retired. He lives at home but poor health has greatly reduced his activity. In the course of our conversation we began to talk about the way one might feel when there are no responsibilities with which to deal. Such a situation might seem quite desirable at first thought. He said, "Sitting still isn't much fun when there is nothing to follow." He had obviously made the personal discovery that, when rest becomes an end rather than a means, much of its significance is lost. Even when health is poor and activity limited, one can challenge oneself mentally and spiritually in such a way as to provide meaning for existence. If you are too tired to run, walk. If you are too sick to walk, think. When you grow too weary to think, pray. Rest is most meaningful when there is a challenge which follows.

Remember the creation account. God sanctified the

sabbath by resting on the seventh day. I also believe that after that day of rest God did not go out of the creating business. His creating has continued right along to this very moment as I write.

A time of rest is not a signal that the game is over. Rest is a time-out for the purpose of taking a deep breath, checking the game plan, and gaining some perspective on the challenge of the moment. We also might conceivably make the discovery that it is not our rest which has lost its meaning but rather our work. The significance of our rest directly parallels the significance of our work.

I knew a lady once who retired very early in life due to a rather sizable inheritance. She considered herself a philosopher and writer. Everyone knew, however, that her occupational identification was a way of having something to write in the blank for an occupation on her IRS return. The lady had about as little to do as anyone I have ever met, but was also unquestionably miserable. She had plenty of time for rest, but there was nothing beyond her rest to give it meaning.

One always trains best when there is a contest to anticipate. When there is no contest, one has little motivation to submit to the discipline required. If one's work has lost its meaning, there is little motivation to submit to the proper rest required to function efficiently.

The purpose of a time-out is to get back into the game and score. Such is the case with rest. Rest also becomes more important as the game becomes more important. And at the risk of sounding like a broken record, rest is more than just moments of inactivity. Genuine rest occurs when one's physiological, emotional, mental, and spiritual dimensions cooperate in such a way that one is refreshed and renewed to give one's very best to one's calling. To envision rest in such a way may give it a very utilitarian role, but such is my observation. Rest is to be claimed, practiced, and appreciated. Ignore the need and discover the feeling of fatigue, frustration, anger, and, oh yes, loneliness. Life deserves better and so do you.